THE

TAI CHI WAY

To Be Healthy & Happy

Dr Paul Lam

Published by:
Wilkinson Publishing Pty Ltd
ACN 006 042 173
Level 4, 2 Collins St Melbourne, Victoria, Australia 3000
Ph: +61 3 9654 5446
www.wilkinsonpublishing.com.au

National Library of Australia Cataloguing-in-Publication entry
Creator: Lam, Paul, author.
Title: The Tai Chi way : to be healthy & happy / Dr Paul Lam.
ISBN: 9781925265262 (paperback)
Subjects: Tai chi. Health.
Dewey Number: 613.7148

Contributing editors: Julie Bawden-Davis, John Walter.
Cover and layout design: Alicia Freile, Tango Media Pty Ltd.
Images provided and used in this book are with the permission of Dr Paul Lam.

A Thank You

I would like to offer a special thanks to John Walter, an experienced USA-based editor, writer and author with a special interest in tai chi. John has participated in my programs at an advanced level and has combined his life-long professional editorial skills with his passion for my tai chi for health vision to make it possible for this version of my memoir to shine.

About The Tai Chi Way

I must be the first person in history to have travelled more than one million miles teaching tai chi, so airports are almost my second home. And airports are a place where one can still find a good supply of books and magazines like this one. In this highly digital world, it is heartening to see that there is still a strong niche for print in our reading lives.

Publisher Michael Wilkinson has helped cultivate this special type of publication though his work at Wilkinson Publishing, and when he approached me about developing my memoir, *Born Strong*, as an easy book format, I was highly intrigued. I imagined the ways that my story about tai chi for health could reach travellers in airports, as well as other busy people passing by newsstands on street corners and in supermarkets and book stores. Although I was concerned initially that an easy book format might duplicate my book-length memoir, my partners in this project convinced me that it is a different kind of work. Thank you to all of them, including Michael, Jess Lomas, John Walter and Julie Bawden-Davis.

Born Strong was written to encourage people to think that no matter how desperate things can seem in one's life, there is always hope. With hard work and love you can overcome almost anything. Tai chi transformed my life and I wanted to share how effective my Tai Chi for Health program has been for so many people around the world. The full-length memoir enabled me to tell that story. This publication does the same, and in an easy-to-read, entertaining way. I hope the reader will find *The Tai Chi Way* to be an enjoyable starting point to a healthier, happier life in this busy and challenging world.

To Aunt, whose unconditional love gave me strength

May 15, 2010: Wellness Day, People's Association Headquarters, Singapore

In the deep of the night, I huddled with Aunt in the cramped storeroom four of us called home since being evicted from the family estate. I tried to close my ears to the jeers and shouts in the courtyard while Aunt anchored me by pulling me even tighter to her skeletal chest. Yet again the Communists had come, bursting into the room after dark and dragging my frail grandmother out into the courtyard for another savage beating. Trapped and powerless in the time of the Midnight Terrors, fear besieged us.

My heart pounded and my palms sweated as the shouting became even louder. With a shock, I snapped back to the present, as I reminded myself that time in China occurred long ago. I stood onstage in Singapore at a huge public event. The shouting came from an excited audience waiting to learn tai chi from me.

I stood on the stage built especially for this Wellness Day occasion as the grand field in front of me brimmed with participants, official photographers, videographers, and TV and newspaper crews. Regaining composure, I welcomed a thunderous cheer from the audience. Two thousand people travelled here to this field in Singapore in the early morning hours to learn from me about the life-altering possibilities of tai chi.

Taking a deep breath, I straightened my posture and put my mind into "upright" awareness, expanding my joints from within and welcoming the energy that coursed through my body. This balancing calmed my mind, putting me in a *jing* state — mindful, serene, in the present. I gestured with my arms to introduce the two CEOs of the People's Association flanking me and Professor Raymond Lau — my colleague, assistant and translator. This action sparked another giant cheer.

Then I led the audience in my warm-up exercises, first walking in place to loosen joints and then standing with feet shoulder width apart. Extending my arms in front of me with palms facing toward me, I brought my hands inches from my face, then turned the palms outward and slowly extended my arms while stretching my neck and shoulders.

As we continued, I shared the moves from my Tai Chi for Arthritis program, always attuned to the crowd, thanks to a skill Aunt taught me as a child. "When you enter a room, Bon Trong," she told me, "you must stop and absorb the mood before you act or react. Only then should you proceed." Unlike the Communist crowd brainwashed by Chairman Mao to beat Grandmother all those years ago, this crowd emanated a profound positive energy that I gladly embraced. My grandmother and aunt would be so proud!

Focusing on tai chi, I cleared my mind, banishing my childhood fears. While my tumultuous early life was a past reality, I remained mindful that for 38 years I introduced people all over the globe to the wonders of tai chi and its ability to improve health and wellness in a wide variety of ways.

My life journey that started with a harrowing childhood in Communist China, though fraught with pain and suffering, brought me to that stage on that particular day. As I looked out at the sea of smiling faces, I knew I had finally reached a place of peace. My calling to share tai chi with others had empowered me to conquer my traumatic past. This was a true miracle, because on many occasions during my young life, it did not appear that I would live very long at all.

Contents

Left Behind
in China

Fortune and flowers do not last forever.

CHINESE PROVERB

My father had to be mistaken the day he named me Bon Trong. Meaning "born to be strong" in Chinese, my given name haunted me for many years. Born in 1948 in Vietnam, the fourth child of Chinese parents, I entered the world happy, but several illnesses lay in wait to claim me during my infancy, including the potentially fatal tentacles of diphtheria.

My father said that I used to laugh happily when he carried me, but then the leading baby killer in that part of the world came to call on my little body, and everything changed. They banished babies with diphtheria to an isolation hospital to eventually perish. No treatment existed back then. But my father refused to give up on me. Instead he kept me home, locating a French doctor who claimed to be able to cure the childhood scourge with a radical new treatment involving administering large injections directly into the lower abdomen.

Despite his meagre wages as an English teacher, my father managed to scrape together enough money for one week of the exorbitantly priced treatment. Right before the money ran out, my fever broke, and I recovered quickly.

My father had no way of knowing at the time, but the "doctor's" sham of a treatment had nothing to do with my recovery. As a matter of fact, I learned years later after my medical training that the injections directly into my abdomen could have perforated my bowel and threatened my life with peritonitis. I am convinced that my father's love and faith saved me.

My time with my father would be limited. When I was ten months old, my mother brought me on a fateful trip to visit my paternal and maternal grandmothers in Southern China. My older brothers and sister also went on the trip and returned to Saigon after the visit finished, but I did not make the return flight.

According to Chinese tradition, in order to ascend to heaven, a direct male relative must see you off at your death ceremony. My father was an only child and lived too far away to take on this responsibility, so my paternal grandmother wanted one of her son's children to see her off to her celestial home. Upon hearing of the request by letter, my father instructed my mother to comply; it was their cultural obligation.

Though they told me later that Grandmother requested that my mother leave behind my next-oldest brother, Bon Quoc ("born to be solid"), to see her off to heaven, Mother didn't want to part with her cute and happy four-year-old, so she had the idea to leave me, her infant son. At first she felt torn over the decision, but the conflict resolved itself when she came to think of my near-death from diphtheria as an omen from the gods that I did not belong to her. Destiny meant for me to belong instead to my grandmother. She took my siblings and returned to Vietnam without me. I would never live with them again.

Since I was less than a year old when she gave me to my grandmother, I didn't consciously remember being left behind, though in later years I wondered why I ended up living with Grandmother. For a long time, I struggled with feelings of abandonment. In true Chinese fashion, I attributed the abandonment to being my fault. As a baby, though, I lived a princely life in Grandmother's house.

A dignified lady of few words, Grandmother carried herself in the style befitting a well-respected Chinese matriarch. She wore her jet-black hair in a classical bun at the nape of her neck; her skin was lustrous porcelain; and she possessed slender, delicately curved eyebrows. Normally stern with others, around me she appeared gentle, smiling, and indulgent.

Grandmother took great pride in keeping her treasured house as spotless as possible. The building was constructed at the rear of the original family house that dated back to about the time that Captain Cook first set eyes on Australia nearly 250 years prior.

Around 1930, my grandfather sent money back home to build a new house in the backyard of the grand old house. Though it took months to travel between China and Vietnam by ship, and the journey proved treacherous, the Lams kept two family homes and lived divided. Most of the family lived in Vietnam where they made their money, but they always had a base in China. So when my grandfather lived in Vietnam, he sent money to care for his wife in China and to build her a new home. By the time I arrived, however, my grandfather had died ten years earlier. According to Chinese tradition, upon his death, his elder brother should take over the care of his brother's family. That meant that during the Japanese invasion in China, my widowed grandmother fled to Vietnam to live with her brother-in-law in 1938, but went back to China as soon as the country defeated Japan in 1946.

Grandmother returned to reign over her new eleven-room home. As for the old house, the family sold much of the structure. They managed to keep the central lounge and a few rooms. In the lounge lay an altar that held ancestral tablets carved with the names of ancestors. There during festive seasons, the family honoured ancestors and made offerings to the gods. Grandmother also used part of the building for storage, including the tiny room off the central lounge that contained a stockpile of rice. No one gave much thought to the room at the time, but it would one day become my universe.

In 1950, our household consisted of my paternal grandmother; Aunt (Ma Xiang); Aunt's adopted son, Ben Zheng; and the young manservant whom we called Little Uncle.

My aunt, Ma Xiang, married my father's cousin at the age of fourteen. The Lam family, like many Chinese families, was very inclusive. My grandfather and his brother treated both families as one. All cousins were ranked and treated as siblings, and the extended family lived in the same house.

Aunt's husband was a gambler and an opium addict before marriage. The parents arranged the marriage hoping the union would transform him, but it did not. As a result, Aunt became the scapegoat for his transgressions, despite the fact that she was still a child and unequipped to control an adult male with two addictions, particularly in an era when women had no rights. Everyone treated her badly, except Grandmother and my father, and things got much worse when her husband died from an overdose at the age of thirty. After his death when the opportunity came along, Aunt gladly opted for the chance to live with Grandmother in China.

A small, delicate lady with gentle features, Aunt spoke softly, moved quietly, and absorbed the mood of others. All those years of living at the bottom of the family taught her survival skills. She learned to anticipate everyone's feel-ings and desires, because she had to please everyone. This responsibility came naturally to Aunt, who epitomised pure kindness. Even at our lowest, most desperate times, she still worried about anyone in trouble, like the beggars on the street, despite the fact that we weren't far removed from them.

Young children possess a sixth sense like animals. They know if people like and care for them. The moment we met, I immediately gravitated to Aunt. Whenever she came near me, I stopped crying, and she lulled me into contentment when she carried me around like her joey (a baby kangaroo inside its mother's pouch). Cousin Zheng, who Aunt adopted at three years old, was fifteen years older than me. He enjoyed hoisting me onto his shoulders and walking me around the village to show off my perpetual smile.

Grandmother treated me like a prince, Aunt gave me unconditional love, Zheng showed me off, and we lived in a beautiful house.

For a moment, life was sweet.

TAI CHI HELPS YOU CHILL

Our modern world has created unbalanced minds and bodies. We experience excess stimulation and stress and are moving too fast. Many people possess sedentary jobs and don't take part in sufficient physical exercise to balance the body. Tai chi builds serenity by offering a slower pace that provides regeneration of energy and relaxation. At the same time, tai chi exercises the entire body, from all muscles and joints to all internal organs and even the mind.

Life with
a Black Label

*A child's life is like a piece of paper on which
every person leaves a mark.*

CHINESE PROVERB

Like the traditional matriarch that she was, Grandmother believed that if you were a good person — charitable and respectful of your elders and authority — you would be treated justly by the gods and the emperor and government. By following that time-honoured rule, she had always gained the respect of everyone around her. And she held her head high because of that respect.

But traditional China was coming undone.

After decisive victories against Chiang Kai-shek's nationalist Kuomintang in the decades-long Chinese civil war, Mao Zedong proclaimed the formation of the People's Republic of China on October 1, 1949, and became chairman. Information travelled slowly in those days, and Chairman Mao's Communist Party of China (CPC) had yet to take control of our part of China. Two months later, when my mother left me with Grandmother and returned to Vietnam, life appeared to be moving along as usual. Mother sailed off with my siblings, content in the knowledge that she fulfilled my grandmother's request for me to see her into the next life. She had no idea that I would fulfil that obligation much sooner than anyone would expect and that she consigned me to a life of hell.

From 1950 through 1951, the CPC implemented the Land Reform Law aimed at redistributing property and wealth amongst the people. Disguised as a high-minded ideal that would deliver Chinese peasants from landowner exploitation, the land reform resulted in bloodshed. CPC party officials travelled to each city, town, and village in the vast country and worked with the locals to identify the so-called "rich" people they believed were exploiting the poor who worked for them. They seized everything from the more well-to-do residents — including homes, money, livestock, tools, and land — and gave it all to the villagers. The officials encouraged public humiliations and executions. The more people denounced others, according to Chairman Mao's plan, the more secure the Communists' rule would be.

It wasn't long before Grandmother was trampled in this stampede of greed.

Our ancestral house had been passed down through the generations and the new house was built with overseas money. My grandfather had also purchased a small plot of land with that same money. According to the strict definitions laid out by the CPC, because Grandfather spent overseas money our family didn't exploit the people. But foxes like Ah Noh (a childhood nickname meaning "little boy") lay in wait, ready to pounce on any opportunity. A farmer who worked the land along with his own, Ah Noh paid us whatever he felt appropriate in rent, which usually amounted to nothing. His demands weren't disputed by two powerless widowed ladies, a teenager, and a two-year-old. With no man to defend Grandmother's house, Ah Noh saw his chance and accused her of exploiting him. Other former friends and neighbours cast their allegiance to her aside for their own prosperity and also rushed in to denounce Grandmother. The CPC then classified us as landlords, and as a result, they seized our plot of land and the houses and their contents and divided our estate among many families, who took possession of our former home.

As "enemies of the people," landlords endured unrelenting persecution and discrimination, and the label would never be removed. We were relegated to live in the rice storage room of the old house. As the head of the family, Grandmother bore the brunt of the punishment. If only it had stopped at eviction. For more than four years, CPC officials forced Grandmother to visit the local Communist office during the day for interrogations, and on many nights the wolves visited our meagre living quarters. Fists pounding on the storeroom door jolted us awake, and they dragged Grandmother into the courtyard outside our room and beat her. When it rained, they commanded her to stand under the junction of the gutters where the water pounded on her back and head until she collapsed.

Other times they pushed Grandmother down to kneel on broken shells. On too many occasions to count, her tormenters, which included former acquaintances, returned her badly injured. Aunt, Cousin Zheng and I had no choice but to huddle in the little storage room, helpless against the brutes who relentlessly tortured a defenceless old lady. During those times of the Midnight Terrors, overwhelming fear seized me. To this day the terror still surfaces on rare occasions, such as when I hear a sudden, unexpected loud noise or I'm wakened from a sound sleep.

I know now that Aunt transported me through those dark days. Living with the oppressive weight of worry and fear, we seldom went outside, except for food and supplies. At the worst of times, I rested my head on her chest and hugged her body, feeling her warmth and love, which made me feel safe and comfortable. She always hugged me during times of stress — like the Midnight Terrors. During those moments in her arms, Aunt was my world — my only love and comfort. Nothing else mattered. Carrying two baskets of needles and threads and other light household items, she rose early each day and went to the market, selling them for miniscule profit. Four years old at the time, I remember excitedly awaiting her return from the market. Every day she brought me something, such as a tiny piece of candy or a preserved olive. I loved my treat, but Aunt's return was the true sunshine of my day.

Though it should have caused Grandmother much pride, what occurred when I started school may have triggered her death. Soon after I turned six, Zheng took me to my first day of school. I remember it being very busy. The school seemed large, with many children running around chasing each other, at least for the first few days. Born early in the year, I was the youngest in my class.

I loved reading even at preschool age, so by the time I entered school, I could read around the third grade level. One day my teacher praised me on my reading skills. By then the other kids knew of my "black label" as a landlord, so they reacted negatively to the praise I received. After class, a couple of kids pushed me to the ground and spat on me, yelling, "You pig! You dirty landlord's kid. You think you are so clever. We will show human garbage who's the boss."

According to Chinese tradition at that time, when one kid bullied another, the parents of the two children would talk, and the bully would be chastised. I went home in tears to tell Grandmother about my altercation.

"Ah B, you must pretend to be dumb. Just stay home," said Grandmother, choking back tears. (My parents were rare Chinese who understood English, which is how I came to be called Ah B. In their Chinese way of pronunciation, B was short for baby, and all children are referred to by their birth order. For instance, my eldest brother is number one B and I am fourth B. Ah is the common beginning of the affectionate way of addressing someone you know well.) I learned to play dumb very quickly. Within seconds I could look like the village idiot, and I mastered various skills to escape notice. Like a wisp of smoke in a windstorm, when necessary I could fade away as if almost never there. I attended school, which was compulsory at the time, but I always went straight home and hid away in our tiny storeroom. I avoided all group activities and sports.

Years later, I realised that because Grandmother asked my parents to leave me behind, she felt the trajectory of my life was her responsibility. While she endured the mental and physical torture, she clung to hope for me and my future. Just about every Chinese parent believes in learning and will do anything for their children to get a good education. The famous proverb in Chinese culture, "In studying books, there is endless gold," was often on Grandmother's mind when I first went to school and before I was pushed down by the black label. This ancient proverb gives hope to Chinese parents, no matter how down and out they are.

What I encountered in school told Grandmother I had no chance of getting a good education or experiencing any future prospects in China. The black label would plague us for life, and we were destined to be among the country's many national scapegoats. This extinguished her last hopes.

At my young age of seven, I didn't understand life and death. Aunt told me that the gods took Grandmother to a faraway place way up in heaven where she would be happy and peaceful. I had heard her beaten since the Land Reform and watched with a heavy heart as her once regal face appeared perpetually ashen and sullen. I felt relief that she would seek refuge with her gods, although I missed her very much.

After Grandmother's departure, Aunt, Cousin Zheng and I lived under constant threat in the small storage room — so close we read each other's thoughts. Any unexpected noise outside or raised voices caused us to jump simultaneously. When one of us felt unwell or uneasy, we all absorbed the discomfort. As a result, we didn't talk much. Aunt would simply glance to one side, intending to get something, like our lone rice bowl. Without saying a word, I would retrieve it, setting it in her hands. And when we needed something outside of the storeroom, such as wood or coal for cooking, Zheng silently slipped out the door, easing it shut behind him.

Aunt always appeared weak and meek, perhaps because she pushed herself to care for me and Cousin Zheng. Though she rarely complained, I knew she suffered from a wide variety of aches and pains, like headaches and back-aches. I responded by doing all that I could at my young age to anticipate her needs and give her some rest, such as cleaning up to save her work. Unconsciously, I longed to find the magic powers to cure her illnesses.

Aunt taught me many life skills, including housework chores like food preparation and cooking. In addition to keeping house, my aunt taught me to use my hands to create. Skilled in handicrafts, she made items from bamboo, wove baskets, crocheted and knitted. When I reached six years old, I began helping her at the market stall.

Excellent at analysing people despite illiteracy, Aunt worked out if they were friend or foe, what they wanted from her, and how to avoid antagonism. I learned this survival skill from her. On many occasions, she explained the world to me so that I wouldn't make any potentially fatal mistakes. This happened when I was eight years old and saw Ah Noh beating his own mother because she wouldn't give him her last possession — a gold ring from his late father. Shocked to see the lady kneeling on the floor begging her son to stop and leave the ring, I ran to Aunt hoping she could help.

"We cannot interfere, Ah B," she whispered, a mixture of worry, fear and pity in her eyes. To get her point across about how we were in no position to help, she told me that Ah Noh had been one of the people who beat Grandmother before her death. "We are lucky that Ah Noh doesn't come to beat us as well," she told me, ending the conversation.

At the time, I didn't know that Ah Noh was just one of many people fuelled to behave barbarically by the Chinese government. The landlord label that Mao Zedong fabricated carried a life sentence for entire families down through generations. The government ensured that just about everything we did — schooling, jobs, travel, marriage — received the black label seal of disapproval. We were often openly called names, like dog, rat, and poison element. The Communists told the peasants who the landlords formerly "oppressed" that they were responsible for correcting and killing us when necessary. If a crime occurred, everyone immediately suspected black label people, who were guilty until proven innocent. Newspapers and official documents stated that black label families were all human garbage.

In contrast to Ah Noh and his mother, Aunt had the support of me and Cousin Zheng. My cousin was a tall, good-looking man. Athletic and strong and an excellent bike rider and swimmer, Zheng spoke well and exuded a natural charm and charisma. He looked so much like Paul Newman that after I escaped China, the first time I saw the American actor in a movie, I thought, *that's Zheng!*

Zheng's biological parents were poor farmers who lived about three miles (five kilometres) away from us. He visited them regularly and took me there many times. They were very kind people, and Zheng could have, like many others, denounced us to give himself political points. Determined to stay with Aunt and support her, Zheng refused to leave, while just about anyone else in the same position would have.

During an official meeting when a local bureaucrat decided to show off just how cruel he could be amidst the mass hysteria that Mao so painstakingly encouraged and cultivated, Zheng received a sledgehammer blow to his skull that nearly killed him. Despite suffering, sacrificing, and nearly dying, Cousin Zheng never wavered in his devotion to Aunt. He lived his entire life treated as a lowly being without any opportunity. What a brave man.

SECRET TO TAI CHI SUCCESS

Over the years I've learned different aspects of tai chi and analysed them all medically — from traditional forms and their martial arts aspects to competition forms. I discovered that the secret to tai chi is the principles. No matter what form and style of tai chi you do, the principles — control of movement, good body structure, your internal state of mind, breathing, weight transference, and situation awareness — are the same. Tai chi principles are the core values derived from the collective wisdom of many tai chi experts. Every single tai chi movement incorporates most, if not all, of the principles, which means a tai chi set, no matter how short, can bring about the full power of tai chi. This is our basis for constructing the Tai Chi for Health programs. We used only twelve Sun style movements for Tai Chi for Arthritis, yet it incorporates all of the tai chi principles and delivers many benefits to the mind and the body in a relatively short period of time.

The Great Famine

Like weather, one's fortune may change
by the evening.
CHINESE PROVERB

Certainly Chairman Mao Zedong couldn't hear the rumbling in my stomach, and he must not have known that someone stole our rice. Otherwise, he would have come to our rescue. I had, after all, squeezed my eyes tight and prayed — his kind face in my mind's eye, asking him for an overflowing bowl of rice and not the mere handful of tiny grains Aunt always made into congee. But even the thin, tasteless porridge seemed like a royal feast now that our ration had been stolen a full five days before we would receive more rice.

Once verdant and lush, the land around us stood consumed. The sky no longer home to birds, the rice paddies and river no longer a haven for the small fish I once walked past, and the land no longer bursting forth with vegetation. As I lay in the still void of the tiny storeroom, my twelve-year-old heart cried as I watched Aunt's skeletal hands check and recheck the bowl where the grains of rice once were. Her eyes darted back and forth from the bowl to my face, as if to weigh the physical toll on me of yet another five days without sustenance.

By the third day without food, my stomach stopped rumbling. I heard only silence as my spirit slipped from my body and began to float. And then Cousin Zheng, who had been out scavenging for food, appeared at the door. "Come, Ah B," he said, putting out a hand to pull me to my feet. "I just found out that Little Uncle works as a cook at a match factory nearby. Remember how he carried you around when you were a small child? Maybe he can help us."

A distant relative sent to Grandmother's household as a young boy to be a servant, Little Uncle became like a member of our family. We called him Little Uncle because he was the youngest of his family. When the Communists took over in 1951 and confiscated our house, they sent Little Uncle back to his parents. Like all of our friends and relatives, he stayed away, but he did care what happened to us. Once in a blue moon, I ran across Little Uncle waiting for me in quiet corners. He'd ask about everyone, and then obviously terrified about being discovered, he would furtively slip me a few dollars, a significant sum for us. Each time he did this, Little Uncle risked getting himself in serious trouble with the Communist government. The money he gave us felt like a gift from Heaven, and our hearts remained warmed for months at his brave generosity.

It had been some time since we'd seen Little Uncle. The CPC moved him to a factory away from our hometown. We didn't know he had returned to the area until Zheng stumbled upon him in the match factory.

On our way to see if Little Uncle could help us, we travelled the dusty streets in silence, knocking quietly on the door of the match factory when we arrived. A kind man with an almost feminine way of moving, Little Uncle greeted us affectionately and ushered us inside, his eyes clouding at the sight of our skeletal appearances. Despite putting himself in danger for helping us, he slipped Zheng a small bag of rice for Aunt. Little Uncle kept me with him, laying my nearly weightless body in a small room next to the kitchen where he resided. I stayed with him for three days while he slipped me spoonfuls of congee until my spirit no longer hovered over my body, but took up residence once again.

At the time, most Chinese suffered from starvation, and rice was more precious than gold. I discovered that like other workplaces, everyone in the match factory brought their own bowls of rice. The cooks added water and steamed the rice bowls in huge factory pans. Like most cooks, Little Uncle took a few grains from each bowl and hid them, which enabled him to save up the little bag of rice he gave to Zheng. He took a huge risk stealing those grains and giving them to us — not to mention how much money he could have gotten for the bag of edible gold on the black market.

I'd been saved from death after all, but by Little Uncle, not Chairman Mao. A brainwashed young boy at the time, I had no idea that as I prayed for salvation, China's dictator led me and millions of his own people to death's door, pushing many through it. Beginning in 1958, Mao's 'Great Leap Forward' became his disastrous and deadly dream to modernise China and hasten the development of agriculture and industry. A genius at military and political strategy, the country's leader had little knowledge of the national economy and pushed his plan despite clear evidence of impending catastrophe. His scheme killed between fifty and seventy million people over a three-year period through starvation and malnutrition.

In his grand plan, Mao sent all of the country's farmers to work in the factories and to build dams and large industrial projects, while he left the women and children to mind the land and gather the harvest. I was eleven years old when the Great Leap Forward began in 1958. I worked in the rice paddies, and like most of the other children and women, in our ignorance we made a mess of the once masterfully managed system, wasting crops and failing to prepare the land for the following year. The hard labour also challenged my malnourished body and underdeveloped bones and joints, later leading to arthritis in my early teens.

Naturally, with the unskilled in charge, food production plummeted. The following year, many of the fields became barren, and the land failed to bear crops. The excellent growing weather of 1959 was followed by a very poor growing year in 1960. Some parts of China experienced floods, while in other growing areas drought became a major problem. Even though we lived in a rice belt, adults and children starved to death in my village — some children because their desperate guardians or parents took their rations. The air hung grey with desperation and no one smiled, except for the few privileged Communist officials and their families. The CPC severely punished numerous people for stealing food. Many people became so desperate for food that they ate soil and died of bowel blockage.

While the women and children worked the fields, the CPC party — which controlled everything including land, tools, animals and people — ordered those men who farmed for decades to work in factories and undertake enormous, impractical projects that ended in disasters and contributed to the collapse of the country's industry.

Our school distilled steel. We took pots and pans from our homes and melted them together with any other scraps we could find in a homemade furnace. This resulted in a grand total of three tiny black metal pieces that we called steel. The Chinese propaganda machine whipped people into a frenzy. The whole school dressed up, beating drums and dancing around in celebration at our "success." We paraded noisily all the way to the local commune headquarters to report the "good news" to the commune boss. Schools all over the country wasted good utensils and immense amounts of time and energy to produce rubbish.

Though hunger weakened Cousin Zheng, Aunt and me, we scouted like vultures for anything edible. One night Aunt awakened me, warning me to be silent. She had a small pot in which she boiled some water and put in pieces of beef. So that no one could smell the food, she closed the one small window of the storeroom and stuffed the door cracks with clothes. Cousin Zheng told us he picked the meat up after it fell off a truck, but years later I realised the impossibility of this occurring during the famine. Zheng knowingly staked his life and stole that piece of meat. The

CPC tortured and killed many for less — especially black label people. That meat tasted so heavenly!

Fortunately, people became more preoccupied with starvation during the famine, so the bullying subsided. We remained black labelled and discriminated against, but experienced no physical abuse, as chronic malnutrition eroded everyone's strength. In the midst of the famine, life seemed so slow and time became irrelevant. We enjoyed no weekends or special days — just unrelenting hunger, exhaustion and lassitude.

My father did send money to us every three months. It proved a difficult task, because Vietnam was a capitalist country then and therefore an enemy of the CPC. No diplomatic ties existed, so money went through a black market. Father would write to tell us he sent thirty vitamin pills, which meant he sent thirty dollars. We wrote back using a ghost-writer to say:

"Thanks very much, my dearest, respected father. Your vitamin pills are very helpful. They saved our lives."

Considering the slick power of Mao's propaganda machine, it's easy to understand why most people outside China didn't realise the truth of failed harvests and starvation. For that reason, I couldn't blame my parents for not knowing how close we were to dying from starvation and not sending more money. Like most of the world, they were blinded to our dire situation.

To this day, I still wonder how we survived the famine. Aunt, Cousin Zheng and I hovered on the precipice of death by starvation for so long that I believe sheer refusal to give in and our love for one another kept us alive. Aunt knew that if she left, with no one to care for me I would soon follow, and I knew she wouldn't live if I died. She quietly gave me some of her food, pushing herself even closer to death. She would and nearly did give her life for me. The bond of love that we clung to kept us both alive.

The disastrous Great Leap Forward seemed to have no end for us, China's powerless and ignorant masses. But by 1960 the situation became so desperate that Mao had no choice but to officially resign as chairman. He remained the country's honorary chair, leaving his moderate colleagues, Zhou Enlai and Deng Xiaoping, Liu Shaoqi, to institute more pragmatic policies.

By 1961 things began to turn around with the new, more realistic and sane management. We noticed a little more food in our rations, and imminent death no longer choked the air around us. As my stomach rumbled a little less often, my mind became even more aware of an unquenched thirst for nourishment.

In 1960 I finished primary school, but because of the cursed black label I was denied entrance to high school. And in China in 1960, we had nothing to do and nowhere to go. This was the Empty Period. There was no newspaper for us and very little for me to read. When I found a scrap of paper, no matter how worn and dirty, I always spread it out and gingerly wiped away dust or dirt so that I could read and reread the words.

We had no plan, no hope, no excitement, no phone, and hardly any friends. Most people turned away from us because they risked being labelled as conspirators.

Like the physical starvation, the mental desert in which I aimlessly wandered back in 1960–62 gnawed at my mind and soul. The human brain needs stimulation. Extreme mental, social and sensory deprivation can lead to severe mental disorders. The social isolation and discrimination we underwent in China felt in many ways worse than the starvation. Studies of primitive tribes show that socially isolated individuals often die or go mad. We experienced all three — social, mental and physical deprivation. The only thing that kept us hanging on was each other. Especially my aunt and me. Her unconditional love gave me my self-worth, and I wouldn't have survived physically or mentally without it.

As the food situation improved and rations increased little by little, the air of death and desperation faded. But great emptiness lingered as I became aware of my hunger for knowledge. I had a great thirst for something to happen and asked myself questions like: "Why am I here? What is life?" The feeling of wasting my life threatened to drown me.

From that long, deep void, something like a seed emerged from nowhere and started to germinate, growing into a burning desire to learn and do something worthwhile. In my subconscious came a fierce outcry. I wanted to live a meaningful life — not just exist. I wanted to bring my beloved aunt a better and healthier life. And I wanted a purpose for my life.

One day in 1962, as I walked aimlessly, I overheard two boys talking about a new high school located in Chaozhou, a city 62 miles (100 kilometres) from home. I caught the gist that contributions from overseas Chinese funded the school and it was open to everyone, especially children with overseas parents like me. I felt like a drowning person suddenly handed a life raft. With great excitement I turned around and quizzed the boys about the school, my mind and body suddenly waking up from the stupor into which I had fallen during those two empty years. I raced back to talk to Aunt, the words spilling out of me as I explained the school the boys described.

"Education is so very important, Ah B. Your father would want you to do this!" she said, catching my excitement. "I will find the money to send you to the school."

Too young and eager to wonder how she would find the money while we still struggled in the very deep waters of debt, I focused my attention on the entrance exam, which was just two weeks away. I borrowed books and studied every waking hour possible — hoping and praying that I would succeed and pass the exam, despite my two empty years.

I couldn't believe that I passed the entrance examination. Soon after, I found myself in boarding school away from Aunt for the first time. Though thrilled to finally have a chance to do something with my life and wanting to make the most out of the opportunity, I missed Aunt terribly.

The newly constructed school consisted of a few small, shabby wooden buildings that included cramped classrooms containing wooden benches, tables where we took notes, and blackboards for the teachers. The other students wore tattered clothing like me, and we each received a small lockable box in which we stored all of our possessions. To fit as many students as possible into the small living quarters, we slept on bunk beds so narrow that turning over in your sleep often sent you toppling to the floor—a rude awakening for those in the top bunks.

The food supply in China continued to improve — meagre, but no longer starvation rations. We brought our own food to school, delivering our bowls containing rice to the cook, who steamed them for us. Aunt gave me a small jar with dry, preserved meat when I came home once a month. On special days, I extracted a small piece of the meat from the treasure jar to top my rice.

Except for living without Aunt, my life was heavenly compared to before. Most of my classmates came from similar backgrounds, so I rarely experienced discrimination and was assessed fairly. Best of all, I truly appreciated learning. I studied every available minute, revelling in the opportunity to exercise my mind.

At home with Aunt, I squinted to read by the dim light of a smelly kerosene lamp, but at school I experienced the luxury of studying after dinner in our classroom under the lit electrical bulb. Looking back, I now see what a blessing the Empty Period was for me. From those years deprived of the opportunity to learn came a consuming yet empowering hunger for knowledge.

Despite the "premium" living conditions at the school, I missed Aunt. When I could afford the bus fare, I looked forward to visiting her, although when I did get home I felt sad to see her weakening and looking sicker and more worried. Aunt refrained from telling me, but I later worked out that my school fees and living expenses must have been a nearly impossible burden for her. How do you borrow more money when you are up to your eyebrows in debt? My guess is that she got most of the funds from a friendly loan shark woman in the neighbourhood.

Then one morning in the middle of my second year in high school, a peculiar feeling told me that something was about to happen. Feeling strangely anxious, I calmed myself by putting my last small piece of salted meat on top of my rice before I took the bowl for steaming. My mouth watered in anticipation of the treat, but I never got to enjoy that meal.

SCIENCE AND TAI CHI

Studying physiology seemed like learning the secret of the universe. I marvelled at the ingenious way the body works, interacts with the environment, self-regulates, maintains itself and self-heals. Like the tai chi world of body, mind and spirit, physiology is the spirit that brought the body and mind together. The beauty of physiology is that once I understood it, I could use the essential principles to work out practically everything. I used physiology during my entire medical career to give my patients better care. Later I applied physiology to all aspects of Tai Chi for Health.

The Quiet Escape

A mountain of knives and a sea of fire.

CHINESE PROVERB

After first period, Cousin Zheng surprised me by appearing outside of my classroom. Because of the long distance and bus fare, he'd never visited me at school before. As soon as Zheng saw me, he grabbed my arm and pulled me into a quiet corner. "Your father sent someone to fetch you to Vietnam," he whispered. "Pack your stuff and don't tell anyone. We are leaving right now. I will tell your teacher there is an urgent matter at home and you have to leave right away."

With all of my possessions located inside the two-by-one-foot storage box, it took only minutes to gather them. I left my blanket and pillow as Zheng instructed, so that people would think I planned to return. As we caught the bus, it felt like a dream. Deep in my heart I didn't believe I would be leaving home and school. Up to that point at the age of sixteen, my whole world consisted of Aunt, the village and school. I'd never known anyone to have left China through the impenetrable Bamboo Curtain.

The trip home seemed to drag on forever, but it only took four hours. After we got off the bus and headed toward the storeroom, it hit me. I would be leaving Aunt. The landscape blurred as my tears began to flow at the thought. Zheng strode ahead at a brisk pace. The excitement he left in his wake soon energised me, so I wiped the tears away and caught up with him.

The idea of leaving China to join my family had always been in the background but never seemed a possibility until four years earlier. In 1961, during the Great Famine, Big Grandmother sent us a message that Aunt Lotus from Vietnam came to Shantou and wanted to see me. The news shocked me. Most overseas Chinese regarded it as a fate worse than death to return and be detained in China.

Aunt Lotus, a family legend, had the reputation of being a kind lady with good business acumen who went out of her way to help others. When her employees were sick, Aunt Lotus nursed them back to health personally. When I met her, I immediately noticed her broad face, prominent chin and kind smile.

"Fourth B, your mum is my best friend," said Aunt Lotus, her eyes twinkling with kindness. "I will treat you like my son." Then she hugged me and kissed my cheek. Her display of affection shocked me, as it clashed with the no-touching, inhibited Chinese way. I recovered quickly, however, letting her warmth and love embrace my heart, where it has stayed.

Aunt Lotus managed to get in and out of China because she went to Cambodia and got a false passport as a Cambodian citizen. At the time, Cambodia was a neutral country with China. She probably obtained the passport through one of the powerful underworld organisations prevalent throughout Southeast Asia. She must have paid a fortune to the organisation, because of the high risk of cutting through the thick and treacherous Bamboo Curtain. Aunt Lotus arrived with a mountain of luggage containing food, clothing and medicine, creating quite a stir amongst the locals. To this day, I have yet to meet someone as outrageously courageous as her. She managed to get safely out of China and went back to advise Father to increase our allowance of "medicine pills". He started sending more money, which improved our conditions and carried us off the precipice of starvation.

Before Aunt Lotus departed, she planted the seeds for my escape — instructions with Aunt to apply for permission for me to leave China to join my parents. Aunt took the necessary steps, but things moved slowly. It took government officials more than a year to reply that since my parents resided overseas, the Chinese government would grant me permission to join them when I turned 21. I could only leave prior to that if one of my parents did the unthinkable and came to China to personally escort me out of the country.

When Aunt Lotus heard about the government's decision regarding my inability to leave China, she approached Father again to remind him of my desperate situation.

"You have to get Fourth *B* out of China now, not when he reaches twenty-one years old, if he survives that long," she told him. "There is no hope or future for him there."

Father offered to pay any amount he could afford, but admitted that he didn't know how to go about extracting me. Headmaster of the most famous English school in

Vietnam at the time, he earned plenty of money. Aunt Lotus responded by digging deep into her connections and went back to the organisation that helped her make the journey to China. They agreed to take on the assignment — a true *Mission: Impossible*. The Chinese government was secretive; it only had diplomatic relationships with a handful of countries outside of the Communist bloc. Traffic through the Bamboo Curtain involved many hazards, and connecting with the Chinese government at any level proved a difficult task.

The underworld organisation devised an ingenious, daring plan. At that time, smuggling was the only way to get someone out of China. Doing so risked the lives of all involved. Their emissary, a Mr. Wu, originally came from China. He had gone to Hong Kong but left behind a wife and child in China and wanted to take them to Hong Kong to live. Mr. Wu needed the money and means to get them out of China, so he worked with the organisation. They bought a passport from a Cambodian Chinese man, took a page out, and replaced it with a false page with Mr. Wu's photo. They gave him a signed letter from my father appointing him as my guardian to take me to Cambodia through Hong Kong.

The whole operation was fraught with danger and uncertainty. We had no way of knowing ahead of time if the CPC would accept a written letter from Father, and Mr. Wu's true identity could be discovered at any point during the journey. When it came to illegal activities like smuggling, the CPC executed people for far less serious infractions.

Fortunately, I was still young and didn't fully understand the danger Mr. Wu, his family and myself would soon face. My most difficult task proved to be saying goodbye — especially to Aunt. When I got home from school, I had two days to get ready. I could see the profound sadness in my aunt's eyes. I knew it would break her heart to part with me, and my own heart ached with an intense pain I had never experienced. When Aunt and I talked during that final time, we discussed everything but our pain. She tried hard to show her happiness for my opportunity, and we never discussed the subject of my returning, because we knew it would be impossible. To leave China was like life and death in those days; no one ever returned to visit.

After I packed, I waited for Mr. Wu on the planned day, my eyes puffy from crying and my heart aching. But he didn't show up. The following day, Mr. Wu's wife said that the CPC jailed him because the police discovered his plan to take me out of the country illegally. She told me to do nothing and wait. After waiting four days, which seemed like ages, Mrs. Wu sent a message to say that Mr. Wu got out of jail and to be ready again the next day.

Mr. Wu had to have an incredibly powerful organisation backing him to still get the permit to take me out of China. It turned out that the organisation had bribed related officials but missed one, so he had arrested Mr. Wu to get his share. As promised, the next day Mr. and Mrs. Wu came with their young daughter and took me. To prevent the word leaking out about my departure, I could only say goodbye to Aunt and the grandmothers.

"I will come back with a big bag of money for you, Aunt," I proclaimed to her, but none of us believed it.

Mr. Wu seemed to be a smart and calm man. Without becoming flustered, he took his wife, child and me to Shenzhen, a tiny fishing village near the Hong Kong border. Shantou is about 310 miles (500 kilometres) from Hong Kong, so it took a full day bus trip to arrive at Shenzhen. When we got to the border, I thought we'd simply cross, since the government officially approved our leaving, but it wasn't that easy. We were required to wait in a tiny hotel prior to crossing because the Hong Kong authority only allowed a few persons a day to cross. I discovered that many people, in fact almost the whole community there, had waited for months, eventually becoming so desperate once their money ran out that they tried to swim to Hong Kong. Escapees caught by Hong Kong police were sent back to China and imprisoned. Those who gave up and returned home to China moved to the bottom of the black label list.

Young and sad about leaving my home, I didn't notice the air of desperation in Shenzhen. Instead, I enjoyed playing with Mr. Wu's daughter and caring for her while Mr. and Mrs. Wu spent time with each other. I also enjoyed the luxury of sleeping on the floor on a foam mattress and using a real toilet. More importantly, we ate great food. Every day the meals contained some meat.

As the time wore on and Mr. Wu tried each day to find a way to get us across the border, his face grew darker with worry. He must have finally received instructions from the organisation, because one day he came back to our room looking relieved. He then took us by bus to Zhuhai and then to Macau by ferry. Macau was a Portuguese colony at the time and less strict than Hong Kong about allowing in immigrants. The organisation made arrangements so that we could uneventfully pass the ferry customs there.

Upon landing, we joined a long queue. Mr. Wu told us to appear nonchalant, but I saw his normally calm face pale and sweating. We seemed to wait in line for ages. When our turn came, an officer grabbed our passports and asked Mr. Wu many questions. He examined our documents for a long time and then escorted us to an enclosed room where we waited as Mr. Wu became more and more nervous. By then, I realised the gravity of the situation and became scared. Were we about to be sent back to China and thrown in jail? My stomach churned and I felt almost unable to hold down my vomit when the door opened and in walked an immigration officer. I didn't know Cantonese, the local dialect then, so I didn't understand what they said. All of a sudden, the officer smiled and handed back our passports. We were free to enter Hong Kong.

The colour rushed back into Mr. Wu's face. He looked like a man previously awaiting a hanging suddenly pardoned. We headed to my uncle's house on the electric tram. I felt weak and nauseous, so we went to ride on the top deck. As we travelled through the city, the unfamiliar motion proved the last straw. I felt ashamed to make a mess, but vomited onto the floor.

Mr. Wu handed me over to my fourth uncle — no doubt with considerable relief on his part. He had been my guardian through the most dangerous time of my life, but I never saw him again.

TAI CHI FOR YOUR WHOLE LIFE

The uniqueness of tai chi comes from its ability to integrate the mind, body and spirit (not in a religious sense, rather the positive inner sense of well-being and harmony). In many sports and types of exercise, people often say you deteriorate after a certain age. For example, in tennis a competitive player is considered old at thirty and performance tends to wane with time. In an art like tai chi that draws from inner wisdom and strength, your life experience augments the depth of the art and your progress is never hindered by age or physical conditions. The more you learn, the more you improve, no matter at what age.

Being a Lotus

*The tree that does not bend with the wind
will be broken by the wind.*

CHINESE PROVERB

A slightly plump, jovial man, my uncle appeared genuinely happy to see me. He took me to his home — a crowded little apartment filled with life in North Point, Hong Kong, where he lived with his wife and four children. Next in rank among the cousins to my father, my uncle was number four, so I called him Fourth Uncle and referred to his wife as Fourth Aunt. A short, attractive lady, Fourth Aunt exuded kindness, as well as great intellect. She had graduated from university — a rare feat in those days for anyone, let alone a woman.

Fourth Aunt helped me through some difficult times as I adjusted to the polar opposite way of life in Hong Kong. Her kindness and understanding allowed me to gain some confidence and comfort. She showed me many skills, such as how to address people, how to relate to others, how to do my homework, about local customs, even how to tie a tie.

When I arrived in Hong Kong, I could only speak the Chaozhounese dialect, not the Cantonese dialect used there. Even though Chaozhounese and Cantonese are spoken within the same province of Guangdong, they are totally different. I couldn't understand a single word of Cantonese. Thanks to patient tutoring from Fourth Aunt, I learned the basics of the new dialect. Everyone in school made fun of my strong accent as I struggled to learn, but Fourth Aunt encouraged me to keep trying and to ignore the remarks. It took a year before I could speak Cantonese and communicate adequately with the locals.

After growing up in a small village in Communist China, moving to this bustling capitalist city sent me into culture shock. I dressed and talked differently and appeared awkward and slow compared to the busy, fast-moving, and efficient Hong Kong residents. A strong discrimination existed among many Hong Kong people against late arrivals from China, even though most residents originally came from China. They looked down on anyone under the influence of Communism.

The local attitude toward Chinese from China proved a worse problem for me than the language barrier. I arrived in Hong Kong brainwashed to remain a loyal Communist. Thinking back now, I realise the absurdity. The CPC deprived us of human rights, our possessions and our house, and my grandmother died from persecution. We narrowly escaped starvation. Yet as a successfully brainwashed loyal Mao follower, I proved to be a slow learner and persisted in feverishly supporting the Communists and adhering to my belief in Communism, which certainly did not endear me to the Hong Kong people.

While escaping Communism gave me a better, more hopeful life in Hong Kong, it turned out that going to

Vietnam was infeasible because the country was at war and I would have been automatically conscripted into military service. So I stayed in Hong Kong and Fourth Aunt found me a nearby school, Ling Nan.

Studies were a struggle at first. Because I didn't know the Cantonese dialect, I couldn't understand at all what occurred in the classroom. Except for mathematics, the curriculum differed greatly from that of China. In many subjects, I had to start at the beginning.

I stayed in Fourth Uncle's apartment for about six months, and had a wonderfully memorable time. My enthusiasm for learning proved insatiable in the new world. I grabbed every opportunity and studied my heart out. After six months at the half-day school, my efforts paid off when I took the entrance examination for Ling Nan. Three hundred applicants vied for just four places, and to my surprise, I got a place.

Ling Nan was a boarding school, which meant leaving Fourth Uncle's lounge and living at the school with other students. The school sat in the middle of the mountains amidst fresh air — a welcome sight for me after months of watching the many people in Hong Kong's busier areas scurry around. A terrace at the school surrounded by green grass overlooked the famous Happy Valley, and a goldfish pond occupied the midway. Every day after dinner, I walked down to admire the goldfish, and then I'd go up to the terrace to enjoy the heavenly sunset. At dawn on the terrace, our headmaster often joined the few of us who admired the sunrise and spoke to us and did his tai chi, which awed me with its grace. Mr. Chin was a legend. He had a PhD in law from the UK and could have been a rich and famous lawyer, but he chose to educate young people.

Tai chi's power and beauty enchanted me as I watched Mr. Chin, who gave me a glimpse of tai chi's ability to offer a quiet oasis that I could take with me anywhere. This experience with tai chi proved far more positive than my first introduction that occurred when I saw a book on tai chi at a bookshop years before. The description of tai chi in the book as incorporating the law of nature fascinated me, but the photos of martial arts applications turned me off. Having been subjected to physical abuse, especially the Midnight Terrors inflicted on my grandmother, I abhor violence. For that reason I put the book down quickly and chose not to read any more about tai chi. At Ling Nan, though, Mr. Chin's introduction to the calming and empowering potential of tai chi resonated with me.

I'd grown up in China, where privacy is non-existent, and then arrived in Hong Kong to live wedged into my uncle's apartment with him, Fourth Aunt, their four kids, and a servant, only to leave and board at Ling Nan with thirty other boys in one room. So it's not surprising that I longed for a bit of my own space. In a daring moment, I wrote to ask Father if he would allow me to rent a small room during the next summer holiday. To my surprise, he said yes, so Fourth Uncle found me a living space.

So small was the room that if I sat on the bed and stretched my arms out to the sides, I touched both walls. I soon discovered that the room was a spare toilet — and

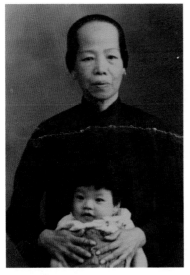

Grandmother and me.

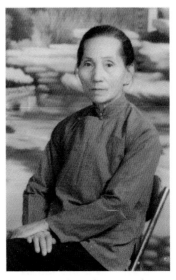

My beloved Aunt (Ma Xiang) sits for a rare photo.

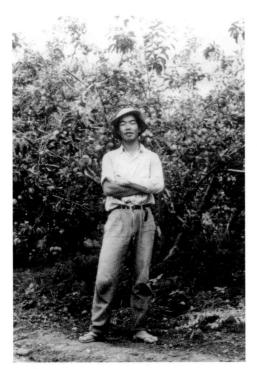

Working at the market garden, 1968. See the two patches on my knees from crawling daily to earn money for university.

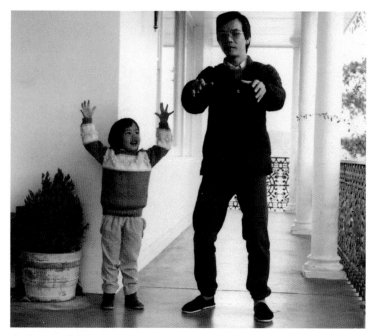

Andrea, my daughter trying out tai chi at 3 years old.

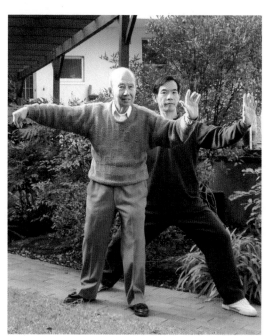

Mr Lum, my father in law and tai chi teacher, in his 90s.

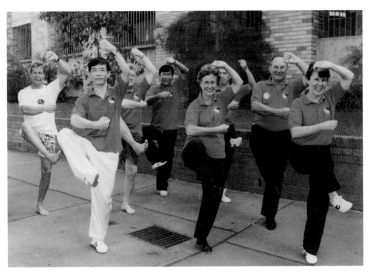

Better Health Tai Chi Chuan instructors, 1989.

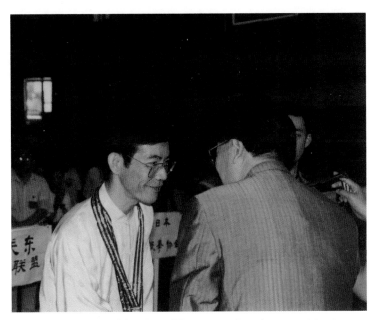

Receiving my gold medal at the 3rd International tai chi competition in Beijing, 1993.

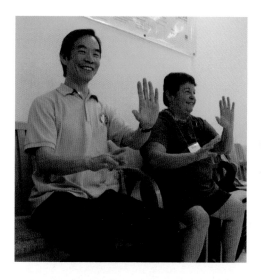

Seated tai chi for arthritis, waving hands posture, Sarasota, Florida, USA, October 2012.

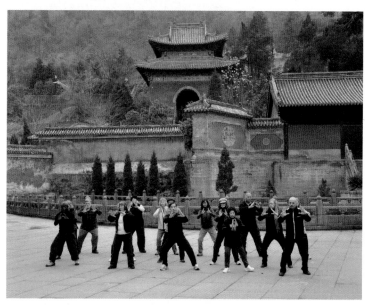

With tai chi colleagues in Wudang Mountain, China, 2010.

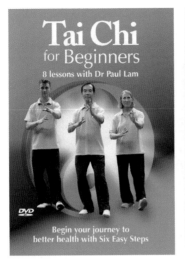

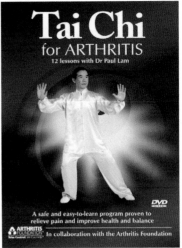

Tai Chi for Beginners DVD cover. Viewed by over 4 million on YouTube.

The cover of *Tai Chi for Arthritis*, recommended by the Arthritis Foundation (both US and Australia) and health departments around the world.

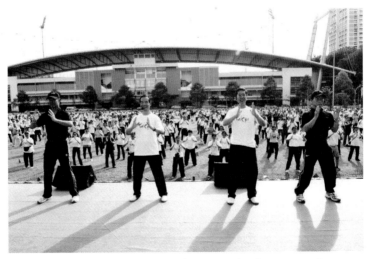

Wellness Day at Singapore's People's Association headquarters teaching 2,000 people Tai Chi for Arthritis, May 2010.

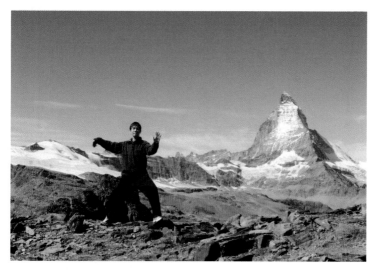

At the Matterhorn in Switzerland, 2010.

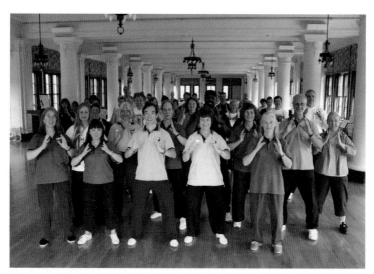

Annual Tai Chi Workshop at Terre Haute, USA, 2007.

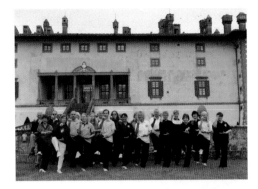

Exploring the Depth of Tai Chi at Artiminos, Italy, 2011.

Accepting the Lorin Prentice Award from Arthritis Foundation of Victoria, 2012.

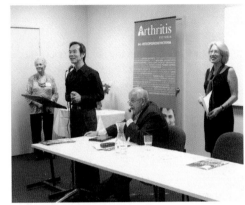

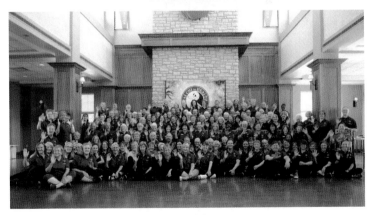

The 28th Annual Tai Chi Workshop, USA, 2014.

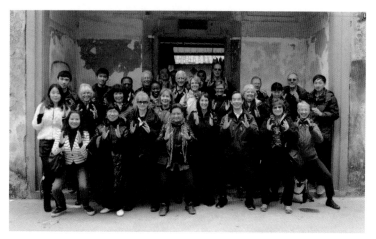

My tai chi friends visited my old home in China with relatives, 2013.

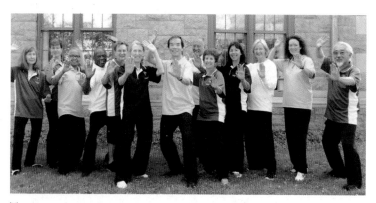

Teaching a Sun style tai chi movement (Fan Back) in Connecticut, USA, 2013.

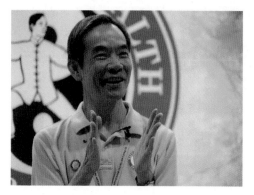

Applauding the performance of my tai chi students and colleagues.

a tiny one at that. But, in that little room I experienced pure bliss. For the first time in my life, when I closed the door, I enjoyed my own totally private world. I spent my happiest times reading. During the days of the August Moon Festival (the most significant festival in China after New Year's), I began reading Louis Cha's martial arts stories until the wee hours of the morning, only to wake up unaware of the time and resume reading. Cha's books tell the stories of fictional martial arts heroes. Usually a man or a beautiful woman with amazing powers and extraordinary martial arts skills, these heroes performed impossible tasks. They went out into the world to right wrongs and save the oppressed and weak.

For the first time in my life during that happy summer holiday, I remained ensconced in my own little world free from discrimination, challenges, and even homework. There in my refuge I read Cha's books and imagined myself as the hero, fighting incredible odds, taking huge risks, and growing in strength so I could right all of the wrongs in the world. I daydreamed about meeting a beautiful lady and becoming a man of respect and helping others.

The next level of dreams was to study overseas, but I discovered that to do so you had to redo the last one or two years of high school. There were only two small universities in Hong Kong, and hardly anyone could get in. If I waited until I graduated from high school in Hong Kong before going overseas to go to university, I would have to do the last two years of high school again. I petitioned my father several times to let me go to Australia before year eleven to study. Finally, upon a recommendation from my second-oldest brother Andrew, who was already studying in Australia, he agreed.

Around the time I prepared to leave Hong Kong, the Cultural Revolution spread its effect throughout Hong Kong and the student movement emerged. Leftist students started to riot, and the situation escalated so quickly that Hong Kong hit a crisis. Housing and share prices plummeted, and many people left because of fear that the Communists would take over.

As it turned out, if I had applied for my student visa a month later, it would have been impossible to get out of Hong Kong. With the mass exodus, the competition would have been so fierce there would have been no way I could compete with my low level of English. I did get out, though I had no idea what to expect of Australia. I only wanted to avoid stepping back. Little did I realise that paradise awaited me.

Falling in Love with Australia

If you get up one more time than you fall,
you will make it through.

CHINESE PROVERB

My excitement about going to Australia outweighed any sadness I had about leaving Hong Kong, and the preparations kept me busy. Saying goodbye was easy, not comparable to when I left China, because that experience meant leaving Aunt and the entire world I knew, and it felt so final. Leaving Hong Kong, where I'd learned to take care of myself, felt like a stepping-stone to a whole new life. I did feel sad saying goodbye to my fourth uncle, aunt and cousins.

On the big day, I boarded the Air New Zealand plane to Sydney, Australia. Everything on the plane seemed so streamlined and sparkling clean. The stewardess served me breakfast on a tidy tray that contained just about any food I could imagine — with some items I couldn't have imagined, like the Corn Flakes box. After careful examination, which included shaking the carton and turning it upside down, I decided that the correct way to consume the contents involved pouring the flakes into a bowl, opening a sachet of jam, spreading it on them, and eating the concoction with a fork.

At the Sydney airport, my brother Andrew greeted me with a hug. He drove me to his home in the western suburbs, a working people's community called Summer Hill where students find the cheapest places to rent.

I stayed with Andrew for a couple of weeks before school started, revelling in the beauty of the land, the clean, fresh air, and the friendly and laid-back people. The polar opposite of Hong Kong with its constant hustle and impatience, Australia exuded happiness and consideration. I immediately fell in love with Sydney and its wonderful people.

Arriving at the Trinity Grammar School as a Year 11 pupil, though, I experienced culture shock again and soon learned that I needed to learn many things in Australia — the most urgent being English. Before I left Hong Kong, Fourth Uncle wrote me a note to carry with me containing some common questions, such as: "Excuse me, sir, can you tell me where the toilet is?" I found that list indispensable.

I didn't realise the challenges of learning the language, however. English is an entirely different language from Chinese, even the names are in reverse order. My name is Lam Bon Trong in Chinese, but in English it is Christian name first, so I became Bon Trong Lam. Wishing to be user-friendly, I chose a Westernised Christian name. I would love to say that I chose Paul because it means "small" or "humble" and is the complete opposite to Bon Trong (meaning "born strong"), but the truth is that I finally found a name I could spell and pronounce with some confidence.

My spirit resonated with the country. I loved being anonymous in Sydney. No more was I a church mouse running across the street as in a Chinese village. I also loved the country feeling in the suburbs where neighbours are always "mates". But mostly I cherished the freedom — to speak, think as you want and plan your life.

However, not knowing English brings so many challenges that even seemingly minor matters can become quite embarrassing. For this reason, to this day I deeply sympathise with new immigrants who lack language skills and knowledge of local etiquette. For example, I suffered through an incident at my school in which I was punished for being unable to understand an arbitrary rule about how to slice my bread.

The incident was minor but a good example of how seemingly small cultural differences can lead to big misunderstandings between people. There are vast differences when it comes to culture and social etiquette between English and Chinese traditions. The tai chi philosophy of listening to others helps bridge the gap between cultural differences and teaches various cultures to learn to understand and tolerate one another. In tai chi we first touch the opponent (or the person with whom we interact) to feel the incoming force before we act. This minimises quick judgment of others based on the colour of skin, social class, sex, or anything else. By listening to the person with whom you interact, you can choose the appropriate response to achieve better harmony between personal relationships.

I found boarding school challenging because of my linguistic barrier and cultural differences. I always missed my aunt, and even more so during challenging times. On November 13, 1967, at midnight in the Trinity High School dormitory, I awoke from a dream about going back to China and found myself sweating with my heart racing. Tears rolled down my cheeks as I got up to write this poem to express my emotion about my aunt.

The memory of my dream (originally written in Chinese — my own translation):

Haunted by the Ghosts of the Past
Trembling with fear
In suffocating darkness
I creep back to my village home
My heart thumps against my ribs
I am frozen between happiness
And dread of what awaits me
Recalling the sadness of parting —
My beloved aunt, the grey hairs, thin and feeble
Ravaged by time and harsh life
A hollow, empty, dark, joyless room
Faint silhouette in the darkness
Holding my breath not daring to stir her
Oh why is she so haggard and haunted?
So many long forlorn days in those cruel years
*   since I left home!*
Tap, a knock on the door
Like thunder, the fearsome heart
Jumps out of my chest

Bleeding, pumping
Cold shiver
In the deep darkness of the night
I wake up to an orchestra of snoring boys in my
school dormitory
Through the mist of tears
Sad eyes in sunken sockets when I left her.

In my dream, I didn't dare wake up my aunt. When I found myself awake at Trinity with my pillow soaked in tears, I lay in the darkness of the night listening to the snoring of thirty boys, infinitely lonely.

After another year of hard study, I was able to win a scholarship to enter medical school at the University of New South Wales. At the combined university admission centre I had debated my choices of study, until a flash of inspiration struck me. Medicine proved the most difficult course to get into; so if I chose medicine and then didn't like it, I could always move over to a science course. But to do it the other way around would be much more difficult.

I handed in my application form and on the way out I saw a notice about a scholarship offered for university students. The program offered only fifteen places in the state of New South Wales. I filled in the form and forgot all about it. To my amazement, I received a scholarship to the University of New South Wales Medical School.

I had made it to the place where I would have some of the most wonderful times of my life.

PROOF OF HEALTH BENEFITS

When I began teaching my Tai Chi for Health program, I observed that many students gained benefits very quickly — sometimes within weeks. These observations were substantiated by the largest study to date of tai chi for arthritis. Led by Professor Leigh Callahan from the University of North Carolina, the research showed significant health benefits for people with all types of arthritis. In the study, presented in 2010, 354 participants were randomly assigned to two groups. The tai chi group received eight weeks of lessons, while the control group waited for tai chi classes. The group performing tai chi experienced significant pain relief, less stiffness, improved balance and better ability to manage daily living. More importantly, subjects felt better about their overall wellness.

A Full Taste
of Freedom

Deep doubts, deep wisdom;
small doubts, little wisdom.

CHINESE PROVERB

As a starving child, I certainly never dreamed about being a doctor. My first encounter with a physician (apart from my infant near-death experience from diphtheria) occurred at five years old. A bicycle ran over me, leaving a small laceration on my left ankle. Cousin Zheng took me to the local hospital. I screamed with fear, so the doctor had four men hold me down so he could stitch up the wound without any local anaesthetic. The experience proved especially painful and frightening. Afterward I had an image of doctors being gods, but malevolent ones to be feared.

My time at the University of New South Wales was one of the most exciting, fun and happy periods of my life. My brother Andrew had left Australia, so I managed myself and had total freedom. Nobody told me what to do, and nobody cared what I did. I went to lectures when I felt like it and I lived in jeans and thongs. I thought girls would not be interested in me, being awkward, bespectacled and skinny — so I decided to be comfortable. Unlike the more fashion-conscious students, I kept my hair long not because it was the "in" thing to do but because I hated getting it cut. I remembered the pain of my early haircuts from the village barber with his blunt clippers. Fortunately, many students had long hair, so I didn't stand out. After being an underdog in my Chinese village, I learned the importance of not standing out in a crowd.

The best part about my early days in Australia was the complete lack of discrimination. No black label or Chinese background like in Hong Kong. At the university, everyone treated me as an adult and simply left me alone. I relished the freedom to be myself. I found a job in a Chinese restaurant and with the money I earned was able to purchase a Mini Moke — a basic car with four metal posts, canvas doors and a roof, with a virtual skeleton of a body. So there I was — working, a set of wheels, a room to myself, and nobody looking at me either the right or the wrong way. It was pure ecstasy.

Then one day lining up for lunch I stood behind a tall Chinese girl, nearly my height, and slim with soft, shiny, long hair. Her back had a beautiful line, and she had an almost rhythmic way of moving. Curious if she was as beautiful from the front, I held my breath when she turned and found myself speechless at her loveliness. Something about her hit me like lightning. I suppose it could be described as love at first sight. It was the most powerful moment I've ever experienced.

Her name was Eunice. She had a beautiful smile and talked softly with a lovely voice. Her manner was quiet, shy and elegant — very feminine. Everything about her charmed me, and I had to pinch myself to be able to converse with her. A first year art student, she was on her way to the city to meet her mother. I promptly ditched my next lecture and offered her a lift, and we made a date to meet on Sunday.

Eunice had a lovely way of emanating shyness that moved me. Quietly beautiful, her eyes spoke, and when she felt happy her voice could melt me anytime. An only child of an upper middle-class family, her parents loved her very much and did everything for her. She went to one of the best English schools in Hong Kong. Possessing a talent for language and interest in voice and music, she spoke excellent English and Cantonese. She also played the piano at a high level, painted beautiful Chinese paintings, and danced and won speech competitions as a schoolgirl.

In many ways, I was quite the opposite of Eunice. I had no talent that I knew of except to work hard. I didn't know much about culture, music or higher-class etiquette, and I spoke poor English. We also had significant personality differences, though in time we learned how to resolve issues.

From the moment I entered the University of New South Wales, life had been a whirlwind. The first half of my second year flew by as I worked 20 hours a week, partied, and spent as much time with Eunice as possible. I don't remember attending many lectures, and I certainly didn't work on anything.

By the middle of the year, I realised that the second year demanded immensely more time and dedication than the first, and I had learned next to nothing. One day, I woke up feeling confused and ignorant, and I knew I had little chance of passing. I hadn't intended to study medicine anyway. I could change to another course and would still be a university graduate like my siblings. So off I went to the university counsellor to discuss how to change my course.

Changing direction would have been easy the first year, but not so the second year. I'd been having fun enjoying my newfound freedom, so who cared if I became a doctor? Perhaps deep down, I never felt good enough to be a doctor, which is why I kept telling myself I didn't intend to study medicine anyway. Better to run back to where I belonged.

The counsellor took my request seriously and called and talked to both the medical and science department heads. To my surprise they said no, I couldn't change courses in the middle of the year. She advised me to have a go. All university counsellors should be like her. It proved the best advice I've ever received.

The Turning Point

After three days without reading,
talk becomes flavourless.
CHINESE PROVERB

I decided that I didn't want to give up, so I went to lectures for a couple of weeks. What a terrible experience. I had no idea what the professors were talking about. Getting up early for a full day of lectures then going to work drained me, so after a week I started cutting back on classes. By the end of the second week, I felt as if I'd never catch up, and I almost decided to give up.

Sometimes in my life, something just happens — like a storm coming from nowhere. Such a storm suddenly hit me and an urge born during the Empty Period to do something with my life overtook me. I realised that it didn't matter whether I stayed or changed course and repeated a year. I hadn't failed the year yet, so I must give it everything I had to avoid failing that year. I'd wasted two years in China without schooling. I couldn't waste any more time.

Once I made that decision, it became easier every day to get up early and work hard. I soon appreciated having a tight schedule and living a useful life. Gradually I began to enjoy the pressure and developed a clear purpose. I knew I had to work smart, not just hard.

As I started to study consistently and with the right methods, I caught up quickly. The complex medical terminology revealed its logic when I spent time learning the fundamentals. I tried to understand the reasons behind everything. Even with dry facts like anatomy, every muscle, artery and vein has a logical reason as to where they are located and their shape, route and position. The entire body works in perfect synergy and with immense complexity. Once you know the rules, you can apply them to everything and soon it all makes sense. Once I really understood how things work, the facts became interesting and downright intriguing.

I found it fascinating to learn that the body works in two systems, internal and external. Biochemistry is the internal on the molecular/cellular level and anatomy is the external. The two are well coordinated and work in harmony, like tai chi. The external shape is the movements and the internal is the mind and energy. When they work together in harmony, the body functions like magic.

By the end of the second year, I passed anatomy. I had a credit for biochemistry. But more importantly, I got interested in medicine. The more I learned about the human body, the more I marvelled at how the body functions and how scientists had come to understand its inner workings. I realised then that I could be a healer and help many people — especially Aunt, if I ever had the chance to see her again. At the beginning of my third year, I started out studying in earnest.

Studying physiology seemed like learning the secret of the universe. I marvelled at the ingenious way the body works, interacts with the environment, self-regulates, maintains itself, and self-heals. Like the tai chi world of body, mind and spirit, physiology is the spirit that brought the body and mind together. The beauty of physiology is that once I understood it, I could use the essential principles to work out practically everything. I used physiology during my entire medical career to give my patients better care. Later I applied physiology to all aspects of Tai Chi for Health.

Psychiatry was another third year subject that I loved, though the school allocated much less time to this area of study. Most medical students are good at math and science but seem to find black and white facts better to work with. We have more difficulty dissecting "grey" areas like the mind, as this organ is extremely complex. You can determine with certainty from a kidney function test if a kidney is failing, but the human mind is mysterious and uncertain.

While physiology is the foundational science of how the body works, psychiatry is the science of how the mind works, and the latter is in many ways more important. Learning both of these subjects helped me to develop myself as a person, care for my patients, and interact with others more effectively. Later on these concepts provided the foundation to create and build my Tai Chi for Health programs.

Add to these subjects a healing, caring attitude and you have the makings of a complete doctor. I've spent thirty years training doctors and I see the importance of this trilogy. The tai chi principles relating to the body and mind are amazingly consistent with physiology and psychology. And the tai chi spirit completes the healing and caring effects of tai chi.

Back in my early teens, I often suffered from pain in my neck, back, hands and feet, especially if I carried anything heavy. I had been doing a lot of physical work since childhood, and since we had no medical care, I learned to tolerate pain well.

By my fourth year at university, my aches and pains worsened, so I consulted an orthopaedic specialist who diagnosed me with osteoarthritis, a progressive condition that he said originated during my teenage years. Prolonged malnutrition during childhood delays the growth of cartilage and poorly developed cartilage does not protect the joints properly. Working with heavy objects also damaged the joints without good cartilage linings to protect them. That's why at such a young age I experienced osteoarthritis, which is often called the "wear and tear" or "degenerative" arthritis.

The specialist didn't seem to be concerned as to why I had developed this condition at such a young age. He seemed in a hurry, so he just gave me a bottle of Indocin (Indomethacin) tablets to take. Indocin is a potent anti-inflammatory that would have eased the pain temporarily, but it does carry serious side effects. So I decided not to take it. Doing nothing, however, the condition continued to deteriorate.

My future of living an active life didn't look very bright. Many people with the same arthritis have hip and knee replacements in their early forties after developing the condition. The resulting pain affected my lifestyle more and more as every year passed.

Though I studied diligently and felt happy with my studies and work, my relationship with Eunice gradually deteriorated. The unhappier we became, the more quiet and dark moods Eunice had and the more irritable I became — which caused us to spiral downward. Instead of finding better ways to communicate, I started smoking.

Experiencing a crisis in my strained relationship with Eunice, I seemed to think that a cigarette dangling from my lips could help solve the problem. When I blew out the smoke, my problems slipped from my mind. The smoke-screen worked liked magic. What's more, it made Eunice unhappy and that seemed to give me a sinister kind of satisfaction.

Smoking made things worse, but it paled in comparison to gambling. Over the years, I often went with a group of friends to the illegal gambling joint in Chinatown. Back then only a few restaurants existed in Chinatown. The gambling joint ran one. It offered the cheapest and best food, so students flocked there. Some of my friends snuck to the back occasionally to play a few games while waiting for their meal. They played pai gow, a fast turnover game with dominoes that involved a combination of luck and skill. Every now and then I put a few dollars next to one of my friend's bets as a show of support. Sometimes I won, which I considered a bonus, but I never really became engaged.

Then one day while in Chinatown, I had nearly one hundred dollars on me — an unusually rich time for me. I felt miserable after an argument with Eunice, so I stopped for a meal and walked into the gambling joint just to forget my troubles. After two hours, I won two hundred dollars. I would have had to work for weeks to make that amount of money. I went home feeling so smart, and my friends envied me.

The cliché of the first lucky win being a bad thing proved true for me — it became a curse. I went back again when things went wrong, and in no time I became hooked. When you are winning, you're no longer downtrodden; you are the king in full control of your kingdom. The urge to gamble mushroomed until nothing else in life mattered. Delirious about big wins, I became desperate to gamble. On the gambling table you feel invincible. Adrenalin rushes through your veins, giving you a euphoric feeling similar to drugs. Time ceases to exist, worries disappear, frustrations vanish and you feel like the master of your life.

Before long I lost what little I possessed. The worst by-product was my loss of self-respect. I borrowed money from friends and from Eunice and then went straight out and lost it all. The debts piled up, and I forgot about my studies. By the later part of fifth year, I had hardly completed any schoolwork. I stayed up all night gambling and smoking instead.

I blamed Eunice for my problems, telling her the frustration from our relationship led me to gambling. Gambling proved so powerful that it threatened to destroy my life. Like an addict who would risk dying of an overdose to get a fix, I had lost interest in normal life.

One day, I came home at five in the morning after gambling away another night and up to my eyebrows in debt. I had borrowed money from everyone I knew — even remotely. At the time I lived in a rundown rental apartment that was probably one of the oldest near the famous Coogee Beach. Rather than go into my rackety apartment that morning, I walked to the beach and sat on some steps. Soon the sun rose, illuminating a beautiful scene that radiated hope and life. Amidst the beauty and warmth of the moment, I thought I saw Aunt standing on the beach. Rather than scold or accuse me, she shook her head gently and looked broken-hearted that I'd turned out like her late husband. With that vision, everything about her flooded back to me — the terrible life she experienced and my dream of bringing her a better life. How did I get so off course and become a hopeless gambler?

Aunt's unconditional love and my dream for her overtook me that morning, and I buried my head in my hands and sobbed. I left the beach determined to quit gambling and did just that. I started going to lectures again and took a job driving taxicabs. For nearly six months until I paid back all of my debts, I worked nightly twelve-hour shifts from 3 p.m. to 3 a.m.

I never returned to gambling, but for a long time the urge lurked inside me. Years later as my tai chi practice deepened — slowly, smoothly and insidiously in the characteristic tai chi way — I knew the gambling bug had been extinguished.

Fortunately, I overcame gambling, salvaged my education and entered the clinical years of my medical studies. We were stationed at St. Vincent's Hospital, where for the first time I started seeing the fascinating part of medicine, when it's actually connected with a real person. For instance, two women of similar ages and sizes walked into the hospital one day with the same problem — a Colles' fracture, which is a broken bone in the hand. One lady appeared to be in agony while the other came in with a smile and not at all distressed. It fascinated me to see how each person made her condition unique.

The mind is so complex. For example, how can a man become so cruel? Why did the peasants beat up my grandmother? Why did Little Uncle take such risks to bring us food and rescue us from starvation? Why did Cousin Zheng give up his life for Aunt?

Initially during my studies, I became frustrated that there weren't clear answers for these questions. It took me many years to see that as an advantage. The complexity and the uncertainty motivate me to learn more and to appreciate the challenge. Like climbing up the tai chi mountain, the key is to enjoy the journey rather than worry about arriving at the top. The more I learned, the better I would enjoy the journey and reach higher levels of knowledge and skills more quickly.

In school I discovered I had an interest in prevention. I wanted to help people like my aunt to build health and wellness from the onset. I also wanted to help prevent people like me from developing arthritis in the first place. I found that I like to understand the root of a problem and tackle it from the start — not just prescribe medication after the damage is done. During the final year, I really felt that with my training I could help people, and I couldn't wait to try all of the tools I'd acquired to do so.

I applied myself diligently and passed my final year. What a tremendous feeling of relief and achievement. I nearly didn't make it, but those six long years had finally come to an end. What a dream. Me a doctor? Now and then I bit my finger to make sure I wasn't dreaming.

My first hospital as a resident intern was the Royal South Sydney Hospital, a small, country-type facility with four resident doctors senior to us four interns. Given the immense responsibility of practicing as a doctor, I felt excited and nervous during my initial days as a resident. We worked hard and shifts were tight. Every third night we had to work through, which meant a full 32 hour shift. And then every third weekend we worked a 56 hour shift, going to work on Saturday morning and finishing on Monday at five p.m. During a fifty-six hour marathon shift you'd be lucky to get a couple of hours of sleep per night.

Despite the exhausting internship, during my residency Eunice and I decided to get married. We had no doubt that we loved each other deeply and wanted to share our lives together. So we took a weekend off to tie the knot. Though arranged hastily and held at a Chinese restaurant, the ceremony turned out lovely. Stunningly beautiful in her wedding gown, Eunice made me feel like the luckiest man in the world.

Then came yet another turning point. One of the most modern and up-to-date facilities in the area, the Prince of

Wales/Prince Henry Hospital, where I also worked during my residency, possessed a state-of-the-art intensive care unit. The machinery of advanced technology is essential for life-saving procedures, but my experience at the unit showed me that I preferred working with people to help them overcome their conditions and avoid getting sick. Unfortunately, a high percentage of the patients in the ICU passed away, which made it a depressing, gloomy place.

After that experience, I'd had enough of hospitals, so I decided to pursue what I love most about medicine — being a family physician. A family doctor is almost like a member of the family. We can conduct ourselves in a quiet, gentle manner and help many people. Back in school, many of my colleagues thought being a family physician (general practitioner in Australia) boring and reserved for the "leftover doctors". I knew I would love the work and find it exciting, though.

I couldn't wait to get started as a general practitioner — but I was not quite ready.

A LITTLE ABOUT YIN AND YANG

Tai chi is created based on the law of nature. The meaning of tai chi is infinity. The ancient Chinese believed that the universe started as a vast void, which is wu ji, then suddenly the infinite universe formed, which is tai chi. This resembles the big bang theory that many scientists currently believe. Everything in the universe is made of yin and yang. They are polar opposites, yet complementary to each other and tend to harmonise with each other. For example: the moon and the sun, softness and hardness, and night and day are yin and yang. They are opposite but complementary, and when yin and yang are in harmony, nature is serene and calm.

The human mind works much like nature. For instance, anger and calm and sadness and happiness are yin and yang. When yin and yang are in harmony, human beings are balanced and healthier in mind and body. Things that are perfectly balanced and in harmony are at peace; being at peace leads naturally to longevity. A well-harmonised person exhibits this balance by his or her tranquility and serenity of mind. However, no one is in perfect balance, just like no one is perfect.

Breaking Through the Bamboo Curtain

One happiness scatters a thousand sorrows.

CHINESE PROVERB

During my internship, the exhaustion resulted in some strange and revealing dreams. One night I woke up from a vivid one about Aunt. In the dream, I saw a deep sadness in her eyes. Sitting up in bed, my heart aching and mind racing, I thought about how I longed to see her. Twelve years before when I left under threat of death, there'd been no hope of ever returning.

But the world had changed. It was 1975, and Mao was very ill. The new leadership was more moderate and encouraged some interaction with the rest of the world. I realised that going back, while still frightening, would no longer be a life-and-death matter. The hope of seeing Aunt again kept me awake that night with excitement. The next morning, I brought the idea of visiting Aunt up with Eunice.

"Oh no, it would be dangerous. I know how much you feel about Aunt but don't take the risk." She looked so worried that I came to my senses and agreed.

But the thought never went away.

The next year Mao died and things looked even more stable in China. I talked with Eunice again. She could see how desperately I wanted to go, so she agreed and insisted on coming with me. I decided to become an Australian citizen before I went, got my passport and visa, and took out a bank loan for the big event.

Despite my longing to see Aunt and the thrill of excitement I felt at the prospect, the fear of the Chinese government remained deep and palpable. I knew being an Australian citizen was no guarantee. As a matter of fact, Chinese officials detained a journalist friend of one of our Prime Ministers for years because he reported about the true China. If they possessed any records of my escape from the country thirteen years before, they could throw me into a cold, dark prison cell and everything I'd achieved, the freedom I enjoyed so much, my friends and love for my wife, and my medical career could all be torn away.

Those who haven't experienced a life under Communist rule may find it hard to understand how fearful and even paranoid people became. In China, if you said something that seemed even vaguely critical of the party, it could land you in jail. A remark, however inoffensive against Mao Zedong, could condemn your whole family to death. My older distant cousin had a schoolteacher friend who, when marking a student's paper, put a red mark through an incorrect answer. The red ink also happened to touch the word "Mao". This slip landed him in serious trouble. He narrowly escaped imprisonment but lost his job and any chance of getting a new one.

I took two week's leave from work, which was all I could afford. When we crossed the Chinese border, it was very quiet, because so few travelled to China. Two stern-faced officials took us into a tiny run-down room for what seemed like ages. Eunice sat next to me feeling anxious and lost, as she didn't understand the official language. I felt like a spy interrogated by the secret police. They wanted to know all about my relatives, including their names, addresses and what they did — basically their entire life histories. Then they wanted to know everything about me, including my family and friends, where I had been every year, and what I did at various specific times.

During the interrogation, the police viewed me with such suspicion that I began to sweat and tremble as I did years before as a child at the mercy of the Communists. I felt just as powerless as then. What if they found out about my escape? All of the horror stories I'd heard about the Cultural Revolution ran through my mind. At long last they cleared us.

Then more fun. We were required to report to the Guangzhou police where we underwent another two hours of similar interrogation. The Guangzhou police eventually gave us permission to go to Shantou — a city close to my aunt's village in the same province of Guangdong. This time around, I no longer sweated with fear. Instead, my frustration mounted. I had already obtained a visa and had full governmental permission to go to my home village, Anbu, so why did they need to interrogate me and require new permissions at every step?

After being made to wait three day to buy plane tickets, we finally arrived in Shantou, where I first had to report to the city police to answer all of the questions again — except these were even more ridiculous and irrelevant. A ferocious policewoman put me through hours of nasty questioning. When she decided to give me an even harder time and demanded that I translate into Chinese all of the street names in Australia where we lived, and in the US where my brothers and sisters had lived, I lost my patience. I'd been in China for four days at that point and though my aunt lived within walking distance, I still hadn't been allowed to see her. My two weeks were quickly running out. At this realisation, for a split second all of my fears evaporated as anger possessed me. I stood up and almost shouted at the ignorant woman, "I can't translate these English names into Chinese. It is not possible. It is a different language. What do you need them for anyway?"

At that point, my cousin Zhi and her husband grabbed me by the sleeves and yanked me down into a chair as they apologised profusely for me. Fortunately, the policewoman seemed to wake up from her stupidity and decided to let it go. Or perhaps sending me to jail threatened to give her an inordinate amount of paperwork.

She stamped my paper and waved me away to go to Anbu, but that wasn't the end of the line yet. Normally, a neighbour overseer would come next to interrogate everyone, but my relatives skipped that step by giving the overseer a gift. After all of the rigmarole — an extremely frustrating entire week wasted on interrogations and senseless delays

— I ended up with only two nights to spend with my aunt.

The anticipation of finally seeing my beloved aunt over-whelmed me when I walked into the village. Before long, just about every kid and some adults in the neighbour-hood followed us — about 50 curious people. So thin were the children, they appeared to be walking skeletons. They looked at Eunice and me with our Western haircuts and clothing as if we were extra-terrestrials. I can still see in my mind's eye the man who rode past on his bicycle and craned his neck so far around to look back at us that he fell off.

Unaware of Western social etiquette, many of the vil-lagers walked right up to us, stared into our faces, and pulled at our clothes. At first Eunice and I felt awkward, but after a while it became annoying and then scary. Privacy was an unknown concept.

By the time I reached the front yard of our little storage room where I had grown up with Aunt, children jammed the entryway. When I finally squeezed into the room filled with wall-to-wall kids, I saw my aunt and experienced the most incredible moment — like in the movie *Ghost* when Sam Wheat is able to return briefly to earth to see his wife. Tears flooded my eyes and my vision blurred. I couldn't see Aunt properly, but I could feel and hear all of the kids pushing and shoving and yelling at each other. Without thinking, I assumed my doctor's voice and shouted, "Kids, get out!" A moment of stunned silence followed, and a few adults (who were not part of our family) looked puzzled. Then I shouted again. With shock on their faces, they ushered the kids out. Finally, we had a little privacy.

When the room cleared and I focused on Aunt, it stunned me to see how tiny she appeared, especially since I'd grown considerably over the thirteen years since leaving. It took both of us a few minutes to adjust and reconnect. Aunt appeared mystified at my transformation. The small, scrawny boy who left her more than a decade before had returned as a much taller, mature man with a beautiful wife. Aunt appeared older and even thinner, with more deep worry lines etched into her face. She wore a shapeless dress that hung on her small frame and initially stood in awkward silence trying to connect with me. Then I motioned for us to sit down. When we did so, all of my pent-up feelings of love overcame me and I addressed her as I'd always done. "Ah Aunt . . . " I said, choking back tears. She smiled and replied, "Ah B, you are so tall." We smiled at each other and instantly slid comfortably back to those days when we depended on each other to live.

Those two precious days flew by as I also met my cousins and saw some of my old classmates. My cousin Zheng still had his beaming smile and Paul Newman's facial features, but the deep lines on his forehead revealed a man with heavy responsibilities. We bought warm clothing for him and his four daughters and wife.

Knowing full well what it was like to starve, I found it especially sad to see the intense hunger of Zheng's malnourished daughters. I was glad to be able to offer them enough food during our visit. We brought with us as much food as we could and also gave them vitamin tablets and money, the latter of which we turned in for food rations.

The unhygienic and poor surroundings greatly shocked Eunice, who had never seen anything like it. After thirteen years away from the extreme poverty, during that first visit I also saw the filth and unhygienic surroundings through different eyes. As I walked the neighbourhood reminiscing, I noticed that the village seemed impossibly dirty and bare. The pond we used for swimming and bathing looked like a cesspit. Desperation hung in the air, like the time of the Great Famine.

We checked into the one and only hotel in the nearest town centre, and it was the worst hotel I have ever seen. The "shower" dribbled cold water and the once-white sheets had browned. The worst was the filthy drinking glass on the table. When I asked the service person to change it I heard her say under her breath, "What do you expect? Clean it yourself."

Though we found the room inhospitable, when Aunt stepped in, her eyes brightened and she exclaimed, "What a beautiful room. Like a palace." That remark hit me hard. How spoiled had I become? Had I forgotten where I came from?

Except for the clothes we wore, Eunice and I gave away just about all of our belongings before we left China. Though I'd finally experienced my dream come true to go home and bring Aunt a better life, I left with a heavy heart as I thought of her and the kids, weak and skinny.

Years later, I would return again. In 1986, I received a letter from my niece in China, Shu Wan, Zheng's eldest daughter. The news sliced through my heart. Aunt suffered from cancer of the oesophagus. I cancelled appointments and got the first air ticket to China.

During the long flight, I felt waves of deep sadness followed by an urgent desire to see if I could do something — anything. When I arrived, Shu Wan told me they'd known about her condition for a while, but Aunt hadn't wanted to worry me.

Aunt still lived in the storage room. When I walked into the dark space, my eyes struggled to adjust as I approached her lying in the shadows. The feeling in the tiny room almost choked me with its desperation, and tears welled up in my eyes as I lifted her bony, cool hand. She looked almost like a shadow. Through my blurred vision, it seemed like we'd returned to the time of the Great Famine, with Aunt skin and bones and struggling to survive starvation.

The next day I took her to the hospital in Shantou, the biggest nearby city with a better medical facility. What a terrible experience. As a physician, I'd heard horror stories of patients in hospitals being treated badly and how unequipped and understaffed hospitals can sometimes be, but those stories paled in comparison to what I experienced in China. The hospital was noisy, unhygienic, unimaginably crowded and hostile.

The doctor showed me Aunt's X-rays and reviewed her case history. She'd been having difficulty swallowing and couldn't afford the hospital fees, so she went to Chinese herbalists and other alternative practitioners for a number of weeks. By the time she received an X-ray, it showed advanced cancer of the oesophagus that had become inoperable and untreatable.

I cursed the gods at the cruelly ironic fate they had dished out to my beloved Aunt! My whole life I desperately wanted to find a better life for her, and I would have done anything for her. I could finally buy her anything she wished to eat, but she could not eat. I am a healer, but I couldn't heal her. Despite my medical degree, I was as powerless as I'd been 22 years before.

I stayed in China as many days as I could at Aunt's side. Frail and weakened from hunger, she sat and gathered all her energy to talk to me. Before I left, I took her thin hand in mine and struggled to hold back my tears. I knew our parting would be absolutely forever this time. Aunt sensed my despair and reassured me, "Ah B, don't worry, there is an experienced, old Chinese doctor in a faraway village. I will go and see him. He will save me. I will be all right."

I can't remember for how long I said nothing, but eventually I regained my composure and replied, "That's a wonderful idea. I'm sure he will be able to help you. Before I go, is there anything I can do for you?"

"Ah," said Aunt, "I'm just a useless old woman. I never did take good care of you. Thank heaven you got out of China in time. Don't worry about me. You are a good man with a kind heart. You have taken care of me and my family. I know you will continue to take care of the children. I am very grateful to you, but I have nothing to repay you. I will return [via reincarnation] to pay you back in my next life."

I wanted to tell her how wrong she was. She had starved herself and saved my life. She made me who I am, and I will forever be in her debt. I longed to insist that she could

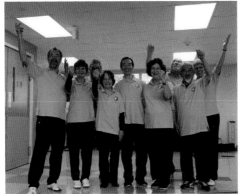

Master class, 2016.

After one of my annual tai chi workshops, Cincinnati, Ohio, USA, with instructor Dan Jones and participant Alice Porte, June 2016.

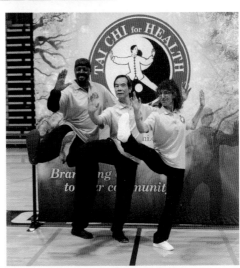

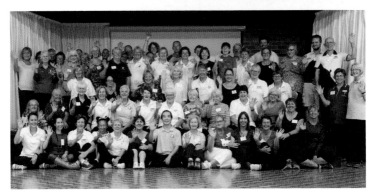

One of the training classes with the New South Wales Health Department, which were offered for more than 13 years.

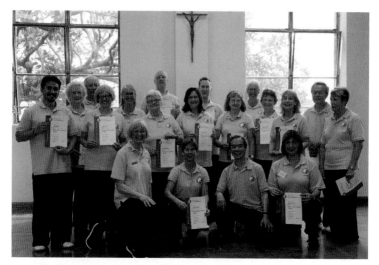

At the Exploring the Depth of Sun Style class, with instructor Fiona Black and all participants, 2016.

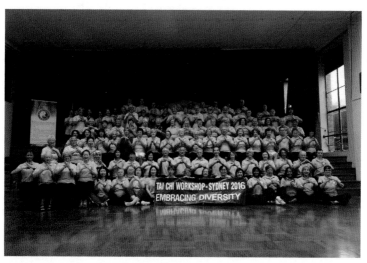

32nd annual tai chi workshop in Sydney.

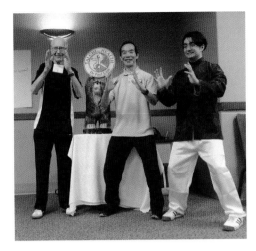

Tai Chi for Energy workshop in Colorado, USA with the youngest, 25-year-old Mohammed and oldest, 92-year-old Lewis, 2014.

Enjoying becoming stronger and more flexible, Sydney, January 2015.

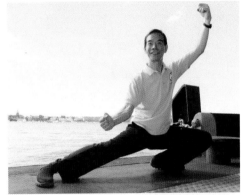

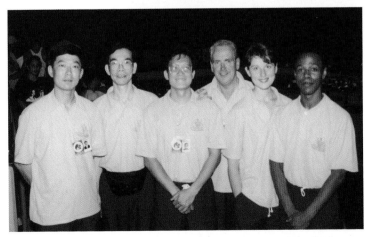

With the Australian team at the World Wushu Championship, 1995.

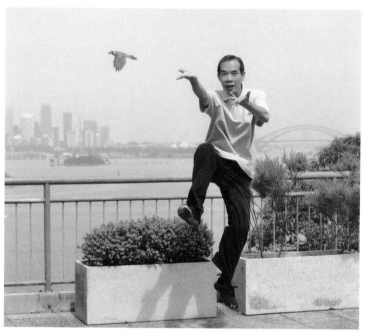

At the 17th annual workshop, jumping up in a tai chi movement to free the bird, 2015.

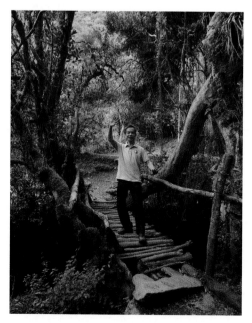

At the Inca Trail to Machu Picchu, 2015.

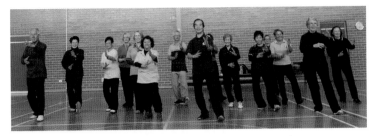

With my tai chi school Better Health Tai Chi Chuan, 2015.

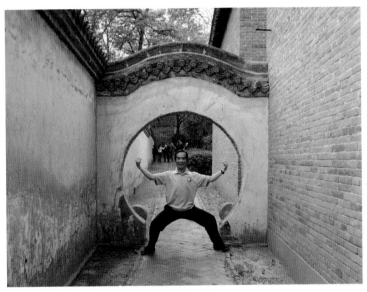

At the Chen village, the origin of tai chi in Henan, China, 2015.

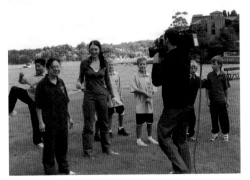

Filming an interview about Tai Chi 4 Kidz with presenter from *Totally Wild* on Channel Ten, 2008.

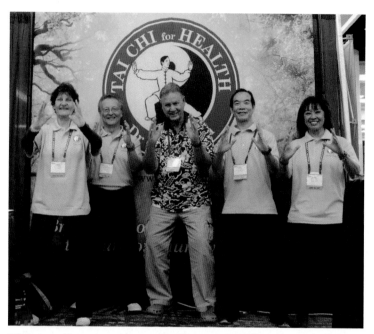

With my colleagues, presenting Tai Chi for Fall Prevention and Health at the American Society of Ageing Conference, 2014.

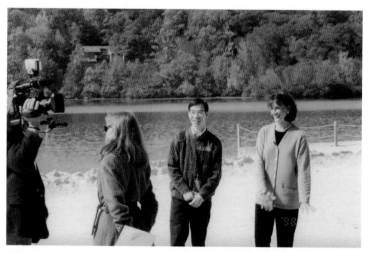

With presenter Dr Nancy Snyderman for ABC TV USA, broadcasted 1998 nationally.

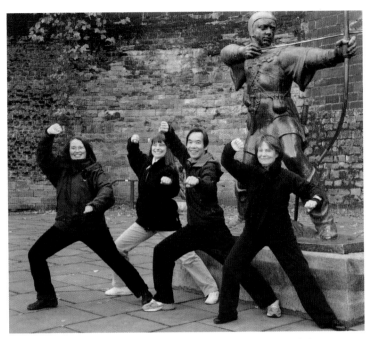

During the Exploring the Depth of Tai Chi for Arthritis workshop in Nottingham, 2010. The Robin Hood statue inspired us to show the "Shooting the Tiger" tai chi pose.

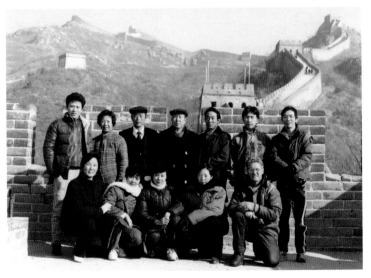

Studying tai chi at the Beijing Sport Institute. I joined the Chinese National filming crew and National champions at the Great Wall, 1986.

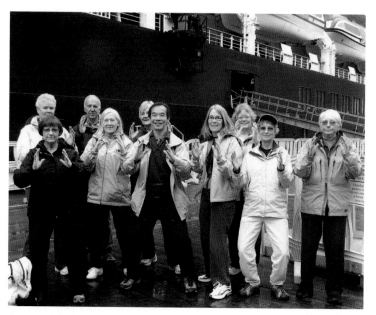

As our cruise ship reached Alaska, my onboard students and I met with local students, 2010.

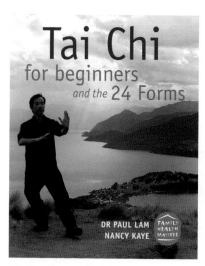

The book cover for *Tai Chi for Beginners and the 24 Forms*.

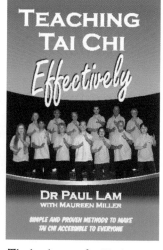

The book cover for *Teaching Tai Chi Effectively*.

never be a useless person and that her love was the greatest gift that any human could give. But I couldn't say anything. I just nodded slowly, in my heart feeling torn.

Aunt sensed my deep pain and sadness about her impending death. She smiled at me, and at that moment I knew she understood what I felt. I could see in her eyes that she would do anything to make me feel better. As always, she didn't care about her life as much as my happiness. Her death approached but the strength in her eyes somehow comforted me, just like how she consoled me as a child.

Aunt died peacefully ten days after I left. I received another letter a month later with photos of the funeral ceremony. For many years after receiving that letter, I avoided grieving the loss of Aunt, as it felt too painful to even think about. In some ways, I'd already mourned her loss when I left China. It took a miracle for the world to change and for us to meet again, so perhaps in my unconscious, I waited for another such miracle.

When I met Dr Pam Kircher while building my Tai Chi for Health program and I read her book on the subject of near-death experiences and how the purpose of our lives is to learn to love, she and her book helped me to grieve for Aunt. I became able to go through the various stages of grief, including denial and anger and letting go without holding back the tears and pain. My family's support greatly helped me in the process of acceptance. Dr Kircher's experience gave me hope that there might be life after this life. I will see Aunt again.

THE POWER FOR HEALING AND WELLNESS

Tai chi is an internal art that integrates mind and body, cultivating internal energy, and promoting health and harmony. The flowing movements of tai chi contain much inner strength, like water flowing in a river. Beneath the tranquil surface there is a current with immense power — the power for healing and wellness.

With consistent practice, people will be able to feel the internal energy (qi), convert it to internal force (jing), and use it to generate more internal energy. This process would greatly enhance tai chi development. After explaining this, I realised the need to show people how to access the qi and jing, so in 2002 I created my "Exploring the Depth of Tai Chi for Arthritis" workshop. It became my most popular, and I've conducted it hundreds of times around the world, with over ten thousand participants. People left with the skills to improve and enjoy their tai chi much more.

A Doctor's Path to Tai Chi

The gem cannot be polished without friction, nor man perfected without trials.

CHINESE PROVERB

I knew that more experience in the family medicine field would make me a better general practitioner (GP), so I started working as a locum (substitute doctor) at various practices. I first took up a locum job in Condobolin, working with Michael Clark, a wonderful GP who loved practicing in a country town.

The practice supplied me with a car and a small apartment. On the second day, my car broke down while on my way to the medical offices. I got out and tried to figure out the trouble when two cars pulled up behind me. The drivers offered to help me. The first one said he'd give me a lift to the medical office and the second said, "I will get the mechanic to take care of the car."

Their friendliness and helpfulness warmed and impressed me, but curiosity prompted me to ask, "How do you know who I am and who owns this car?"

"Everyone in town knows a new doctor is here," one of the men said.

While I liked being recognised and appreciated the help, I also felt uncomfortable at his remark. Then I realised that my mind had transported me back to my village — the country town where everyone denigrated us as a landlord family and forced us to hide in the little storeroom. I realised then why I enjoyed the anonymity of cities. Even though on a conscious level I knew my experience as a country GP couldn't compare to China, that incident made being a GP in a small town less attractive.

I greatly enjoyed working in the country, finding it fulfilling and educational. Michael asked me to join the practice on my second day at work, and while the offer tempted me I also knew that Michael's wife found the small town life challenging. I thought of Eunice, who loves art and culture, and how she might have the same challenges as Mrs. Clark, so I turned down his offer.

After graduating from medical school, my arthritis worsened. My first trip to the Thredbo ski resort revealed what the future had in store for me. After only a couple of hours of skiing, my pain ran deep. By the time I got home, I could hardly walk or move.

It took many weeks to downsize from the severe aches and pains to the usual daily discomfort. The experience showed me how bad my arthritis had become and that I had to do something about it. I recalled hearing years before in my village in China that tai chi helped arthritis. I also recalled the headmaster at Ling Nan, Mr. Chin, doing tai chi at sunrise every morning. I decided to give it a try and started looking for a teacher.

Back in 1976, finding a tai chi teacher proved difficult. I went to one teacher's class, who taught me the classical Yang style and Push Hands. I didn't feel right about him, though. He had a nervous, jittery way of talking and moving that didn't seem consistent with my image of a tai chi practitioner. His dirty fingernails also bothered me, but I didn't decide to stop practicing with him until my father-in-law, Mr. Lum Wan Kwai, told my wife that the teacher was not a good tai chi practitioner. I respected my father-in-law's judgment and went looking for another teacher.

I met another teacher, an engineer and very nice man with clean fingernails. He told me about his tai chi journey. He had learned a variation of the Yang style from a famous tai chi master, who placed much emphasis on relaxation. He invited me to his class where I saw that many of his students closed their eyes and assumed hunched postures, moving about almost formlessly. That didn't look right to me either. I debated about whether to join his class when my wife told me that her father said he was no good either. Then I got curious and asked Eunice what her father knew about tai chi. She told me that he had practiced tai chi since her childhood and had studied under a famous teacher, so I asked if Eunice's father would teach me.

My late father-in-law was one of the nicest and most unassuming men I have ever met. Born in Australia and educated in Hong Kong, he later married and lived in Hong Kong for many years. He and I share similar backgrounds. Like me, he had ties to China and grew up without his parents. His father died when he was just a baby and his mother put him in boarding school and didn't seem very interested in him.

So modest was Mr. Lum that he had never told me — but I later found out — that his teacher, Yang Shou-zhong, was hailed as one of the most famous, if not the most famous, tai chi masters in the world. Yang Shou-zhong was the eldest son of Yang Cheng-fu, the grandson of the creator of the Yang style tai chi. Among the many styles of tai chi, Yang is by far the most popular. The tai chi world regarded Yang Cheng-Fu as the father of modern tai chi, as he brought the practice to many people in China in the 19th century. My father-in-law and his friends were Yang Shou-zhong's first group of students. Together a few of them paid for the down payment on Yang Shou-zhong's apartment. As a result, this group benefited from special teaching from the great master.

Yang Shou-zhong taught my father-in-law personally for years until Mr. Lum moved from Hong Kong to his birthplace in Australia. During our tai chi lessons, my father-in-law told me a great deal about Yang, including his personality, power and mannerisms. For example, the tai chi master took small, almost measured steps when he walked and he possessed a seemingly unlimited capacity for food and alcohol, yet kept a slim figure.

At the time of my lessons, Mr. Lum was in his late sixties and retired, but he looked much younger than his years. Slim, agile, and shorter than me, he possessed the skin of a twenty-year-old. Like a Chinese scholar, he exuded a gentle and learned manner. He shared his knowledge without reservation. Three times a week I visited my father-in-law's small lounge where he gave me lessons. Mr. Lum was soft-spoken and moved slowly and gently yet exuded an inner power that I didn't understand then, but could feel. I would try to imitate him, but I only managed to do the movements without the power. Every once in a while, he offered corrections, but he seldom checked my progress or offered praise.

Mr. Lum was fond of telling me about the inner powers of the great master Yang. For example, I learned that at the practice drill of Pushing Hands, when two people push each other to experience the opposite force, Mr. Yang would suddenly push a student's feet away with a subtle, almost invisible movement that sent the student back as though pushed by an immense force. But he always ensured that the student fell back toward a safe space and grasped him before he fell. Yang focused on internal energy (*qi*) and force (*jing*), yet only on rare occasions and only to his close students explained how to generate inner energy and internal force.

I learned the entire classical Yang 108 Forms and I kept coming back for more tea, corrections, practices together and questions and answers. I felt very fortunate to have the opportunity to learn from my father-in-law, and the teaching of Master Yang through him. What a gift to be able to learn from such a close link to the creator of the most popular tai chi style.

I especially enjoyed discovering how the ancient practice benefits your mind. The uniqueness of tai chi comes from its ability to integrate the mind, body and spirit (not in a religious sense, rather the positive inner sense of well-being and harmony). In many sports and types of exercise, people often say you deteriorate after a certain age. For example, in tennis a competitive player is considered old at thirty and performance tends to wane with time. In an art like tai chi that draws from inner wisdom and strength, your life experience augments the depth of the art and your progress is never hindered by age or physical conditions. The more you learn, the more you improve, no matter what age.

As I progressed in tai chi, Mr. Lum encouraged me to expand my horizons and learn other forms and styles. In this regard, he was highly unconventional. Traditional tai chi teachers often insist on absolute loyalty. Later when I began teaching tai chi, one of my workshop participants told me her teacher expelled her from his school because she studied my instructional DVD.

The benefits of tai chi did not come easily to me. Years of malnutrition and emotional abuse had significantly weakened my physical condition. Prior to studying tai chi, I had thought myself uncoordinated and poor at any sports. I needed to work much harder than other practitioners in order to gain the same level of fitness. I practiced regularly and made progress, however my poor immunity caused me to develop a viral infection every time I reached a slightly higher level of fitness, and that would set me back again.

Later on when I began teaching my Tai Chi for Health program, I observed that many students gained benefits very quickly — sometimes within weeks. These observations were substantiated by the largest study to date of Tai Chi for Arthritis. Led by Professor Leigh Callahan from the University of North Carolina, the research showed significant health benefits for people with all types of arthritis. In the study, presented in 2010, 354 participants were randomly assigned to two groups. The tai chi group received eight weeks of lessons, while the control group waited for tai chi classes. The group performing tai chi experienced significant pain relief, less stiffness, improved balance and better ability to manage daily living. More importantly, subjects felt better about their overall wellness.

I constructed my programs specifically to improve health and wellness. Many other medical and tai chi experts further enhanced them. The tai chi I originally practiced with Mr. Lum represented the traditional tai chi taught by people who didn't understand medical conditions. That is another important reason it took me so long to gain the same health benefits.

Despite the challenges back then, I persevered at learning tai chi. By the second year, I noticed my pain had subsided, and I had developed increased muscle strength. I could hold my doctor's bag and do house calls without problems. I also came down with fewer upper respiratory tract infections. Before tai chi, I got sick every two weeks, catching every cold and flu bug from my patients. It took me a week or two to recover, and then I picked up a new bug. After several years studying tai chi, I noticed that I became sick much less often, and by the ten-year mark I hardly ever got a cold or flu.

The most powerful effects of tai chi for me were the mental strength, confidence, serenity and intrinsic joy that practicing gave me. As I grew with my tai chi practice and reached more advanced levels, I incorporated the tai chi principles into my daily life. I became more mindful of my emotional state and better able to manage it. As I learned to accept, cherish and improve myself, I used that skill to interact with others. I became able to absorb and redirect incoming forces — especially angry ones, which enabled me to help my patients, friends, family and tai chi colleagues to develop their inner strength.

I started my medical practice squatting, which means starting from ground zero. In Australia, you aren't allowed to advertise medical practices, so it can take a long time for patients to find you. The first day that I opened in the small Sydney suburb of Narwee, two people wandered in, but the second day nobody came. The word did get out, however, so I gradually got patients.

I practiced in a conservative area, and the people didn't like change. Initially, only those unable to get an appointment with their regular doctor came to me. They would ask apologetically, "Do you mind seeing my son, Johnnie? He is very sick, and we cannot get an appointment with our usual doctor."

Like my aunt, who could stop a baby from crying in an instant and to whom all of the neighbourhood children flocked, I know how to get along with kids. Many parents marvelled at how the kids stopped crying when they walked into my consultation room, which made my chest swell with pride. Parents who brought their children to see me when their doctor couldn't see them would often return and tell me, "Sorry, Doctor. Johnnie only wants to see you.

He refused to see our other doctor." Eventually, the adults switched to my practice, too.

As soon as my practice became established, we decided it was time to have a family. I was overjoyed when Eunice became pregnant with our first child. It turned out to be a son, who we named Matthew Wei-Sun Lam. In Chinese, "Wei-Sun" means "great life". Our beautiful boy, who possessed a happy and contented nature, enchanted us. I worked long hours, leaving home at eight-thirty in the morning and sometimes not returning until nine at night. No matter how late I got home, I loved taking care of Matthew, bathing him and changing his nappy. He stayed awake until I got home to bathe him and put him to bed. No matter how stressful my day was, seeing my son's smiling face made me indescribably happy.

About three and a half years later, Eunice gave birth to our daughter, Andrea. Our children looked almost identical as babies, but they grew into two very different people — in looks, behaviour, interests and so many other things. Most importantly, they are great "mates", which means so much to both of us, who grew up without siblings. I often carried both Matthew and Andrea, one on each arm, and felt an overwhelming sensation of our love and energy as one.

Even more important than developing my practice, tai chi and myself, I did everything possible to help my children develop as they grew. Matthew and Andrea are the most wonderful gifts of my life. I loved watching and helping my children grow and mature and sharing in their happiness and when necessary, their pain.

CLIMBING THE TAI CHI MOUNTAIN

I distilled the essential tai chi principles from many years of studies and practice and translated them into plain language that focuses on the body's internal components, structure and outward movements. Song and jing are the key internal components. Song refers to loosening or gently expanding from within all joints. This loosening then leads to strengthening the joints and relaxation of the mind. Jing, when used with tai chi, represents mental quietness or serenity and being mindful of the present. Both song and jing are most powerful at cultivating qi.

The body structure consists of correct alignment and weight transfer. Controlling all tai chi movements to be slow, smooth and continuous stretches and exercises the entire body and enhances the jing and song. Moving gently against mild resistance develops internal strength.

Translating the principles into easy-to-understand language and practical movements allows participants to experience them. All principles have many layers of depth and as we climb the tai chi mountain, the air gets fresher and the view more beautiful.

The Spirit of Competition

*Teachers open the door, but you must
enter by yourself.*

CHINESE PROVERB

In 1995 I began seeking a partner to share the over-whelming patient load and to enable me to spend more time with my family and on tai chi. I asked one of my best trainee registrars to join my practice. A foreign graduate from the Philippines who worked in that country prior, Dr Richard Cue was well liked by our patients. I appreciated his gentle manner, life experience and caring attitude, so I invited him to be my partner. It turned out to be a great decision. We worked very well together and he never once complained when I walked into his office and announced that I would be taking two months off to teach tai chi. From 2000, I began teaching tai chi for six months out of each year, and I could never have done that without his help.

My study at the time included psychology — Freud, Beck's *Cognitive Therapy* and Glasser's *Choice Theory*. I learned much from great thinkers and researchers like Stephen Covey, Martin Seligman (leader in positive psychology well shown in his book *Flourish*) and Mihaly

Csikszentmihalyi (leader of studies on flow). They are brilliant explorers of the mind who often couple their theories with ingenious research that shows how individuals develop themselves personally and achieve greater life fulfilment. The more I studied these theories, the more surprised I became at the similarities between self-growth concepts and tai chi principles.

Tai chi is created based on the law of nature. The meaning of tai chi is infinity. The ancient Chinese believed that the universe started as a vast void, which is *wu ji*, then suddenly the infinite universe formed, which is tai chi. This resembles the big bang theory that many scientists currently believe. Everything in the universe is made of yin and yang. They are polar opposites, yet complementary and tend to harmonise with each other. For example: the moon and the sun, softness and hardness, and night and day are yin and yang. They are opposite but complementary, and when yin and yang are in harmony, nature is serene and calm.

The human mind works much like nature. For instance, anger and calm and sadness and happiness are yin and yang. When yin and yang are in harmony, human beings are balanced and healthier in mind and body. Things that are perfectly balanced and in harmony are at peace; being at peace leads naturally to longevity. A well-harmonised person exhibits this balance by his or her tranquillity and serenity of mind. However, no one is in perfect balance, just like no one is perfect.

Our modern world has created unbalanced minds and bodies. We experience excess stimulation and stress and are moving too fast. Many people possess sedentary jobs and don't take part in sufficient physical exercise to balance the body. Tai chi builds serenity by offering a slower pace that provides regeneration of energy and relaxation. At the same time, tai chi exercises the entire body, from all muscles and joints to all internal organs and even the mind.

The philosophy of tai chi's martial arts application proved revolutionary in its time. It didn't encourage fighting blow to blow and blocking and hitting back harder to win over your opponent. The ultimate purpose was to harmonise with your opponent. Tai chi movement does not start with aggressive attack, rather with listening to the incoming force, yielding, absorbing and redirecting that force, and utilising the incoming with your own force to reach harmony. During my years in practice, as I personally discovered the many benefits of tai chi, I started recommending that my patients give it a go. One of my patients and a good friend, Scottie Porter, had arthritis, so I sent him off to learn tai chi. A year later he came in for a check-up. I asked him about his tai chi progress, and he complained about the difficulty he had with the teacher, especially with the fact that what the teacher instructed him to do worsened his condition. Out of the blue, I heard myself saying, "Come to my house. I will give you some lessons."

After a few months of private lessons, Scottie encouraged me to start a school. Knowing my busy schedule, he offered to do all of the organising work, leaving the teaching to me. That proved to be an offer I couldn't refuse.

We named the school Better Health Tai Chi Chuan after the full Chinese name for tai chi. My first class had eight students, all of whom joined from word of mouth. In time, many of my patients would join. We practiced diligently and quietly, working on improving ourselves but never worrying about expanding the school or making money.

Soon I would have the good fortune of working with my friend Ling Wong in San Francisco. Ling has practiced tai chi and martial arts since childhood. He told me about his brilliant teacher, Professor Men Hui Feng. I wrote to Professor Men and his wife, Professor Kan Gui Xiang, both teachers at the Beijing Institute of Physical Education and the most famous tai chi teachers in the world. Fond of Ling, they responded quickly and encouraged me to visit them. I got a bank loan to make a trip to Beijing to train with them.

When I first met Professor Men, he asked what tai chi form I wanted to learn, and I told him I preferred the traditional Yang taught by my father-in-law. I commented that if he could improve upon that style, I'd appreciate it. He said, "Show me." So right there on the street on an empty corner, he squatted down and watched me do my Yang style form. After I finished, he said, "Oh . . ."

The blank look on his face made me recall Chinese tradition and custom. Traditional tai chi teachers don't focus on what the student wants. The teacher teaches whatever he or she wishes to teach, and the student must accept it wholeheartedly. I realised at Professor Men's reaction that he expected me to follow his lead. At the time, China had just opened up to the outside world. Professor Men had probably heard that overseas teachers were more student-orientated, so he asked me what I wanted to learn out of politeness, but when I actually told him what I wanted, he didn't know how to respond to my request.

I knew what I had to do, so I said, "Professor Men, I am here to learn. Whatever you wish to teach me, I will be honoured."

After that, whenever in Beijing, I switched from a Western mode to a subservient Chinese manner. That meant absolute, unquestioning obedience to my teachers. Often close students take care of their teachers' personal needs, like my father-in-law who paid a significant sum for his teacher's apartment. I did my part by giving my Chinese professors as much of my personal income as I could.

In Beijing, I learned various styles of tai chi and a different approach and focus. They placed great emphasis on competition. With competitions, aesthetic value is crucial. At first I didn't care too much about the external aspects, as tai chi is an internal art, which is what attracted me to the practice in the first place. However, I'd already made the decision to follow the teachers' instructions totally, so I did.

With diligent work, I learned many different sets of tai chi, including the most popular 24 Forms, the Combined 42 Form, the Combined 48 Form, the Sun style 73 Form, the Chen 36 and 56, and the several sets of sword forms. The depth of tai chi, however, came after a long time of diligent and continual practice. The key to tai chi is the true understanding of the principles common to all styles and forms.

And that understanding only comes with sound knowledge and consistent, mindful practice.

One day Professor Men said to me, "Paul, you should enter the 1993 International Tai Chi Competition in Beijing." It was the busiest season for my medical practice, with two young children and a heavy mortgage I could ill afford to take two weeks off to go. I also wanted to say that I am not a competitive person. But I complied like a typical Chinese student.

We went a week in advance to train. Competitors were allowed to enter a maximum of three events, and I chose the Combined 42 Forms, the 42 Sword Form and the Chen style 36 Form — three of the most intensely competed sets. I had no idea if I would qualify to enter the competition in these sets; I only chose these forms because I liked them. Winning hadn't entered my mind. I took a team from our school that chose different sets, like me based totally on personal preference.

At 45, I was one of the oldest competitors. A mature category for those over 40 existed, but my teacher wanted me to be at the main events. I had no idea of my chances and didn't care about winning, so it didn't faze me to compete against younger, professional tai chi practitioners and athletes.

I urged my team to take advantage of the opportunity to train with the excellent teachers, never mind winning or losing. Having decided that, and as I continued to train hard, something uncomfortable started sneaking into my head. I started thinking more seriously about injuries and about my fellow team members. The training we did, especially for the competition, put a great emphasis on lowering the stance. This meant stretching to your limit, and sometimes past, which could lead to injury.

At that point, I reviewed my real purpose of my tai chi journey. I started tai chi as a way to help manage my arthritis. As that became well managed, I enjoyed it so much that I allowed my approach and goal to change. The competition's increased potential of injury stood directly opposed to my original goal of health and harmony. Putting all that aside, however, I pressed on with my training.

Like the Olympics, the ceremony and atmosphere inspired awe. The mayor of Beijing opened the ceremony, and a full military band played. There were more than thirty countries represented, all marching under huge banners announcing their homelands. As we entered the arena, with the band playing and the spectators cheering, it felt electrifying. We brimmed with pride at representing Australia.

So excited were we to be at the competition that our team won several silver and bronze medals. I won the gold for the Combined 42 Forms and silver for the Chen 36 Forms and the Combined 42 Sword Forms, and had the highest total score.

The medal presentation and the closing ceremony were incredibly exciting, especially considering my surprise at winning. At the conclusion of the Olympics-style ceremony, all of the gold medal winners demonstrated our winning forms. The euphoria from the entire experience infected me with the competition bug.

FINDING HARMONY IN RELATIONSHIPS

The tai chi philosophy of listening to others helps bridge the gap between cultural differences and teaches various cultures to learn to understand and tolerate one another. In tai chi we first touch the opponent (or the person with whom we interact) to feel the incoming force before we act. This minimises quick judgment of others based on the colour of skin, social class, sex or anything else. By listening to the person with whom you interact, you can choose the appropriate response to achieve better harmony in personal relationships.

Climbing
the Tai Chi
Mountain

*Do not fear going forward slowly; fear only
to stand still.*

CHINESE PROVERB

We came home to Australia from the tai chi competition to a heroes' welcome. I proceeded to push aside the uneasy feeling about injuries and focused on promoting tai chi through competitions. At that stage I didn't yet have a clear distinction between the traditional tai chi and what would later become my Tai Chi for Health program. My intention at that time was to spread the word about tai chi, since it had benefited me so much. Later I saw the need for creating special programs based on traditional, authentic tai chi that incorporated modernised medical knowledge and current teaching methods.

With my encouragement and training, many of my students competed, and a number of them represented Australia in national and international competitions and won many medals. Because of our students' involvement in competing, I joined various martial arts organisations and judging panels to promote competitions within Australia and internationally. I accepted the positions with the aim of steering the competitions toward the internal aspects of tai chi.

A few years went by and I started to see things more clearly. The emphasis for the competitions was on aesthetics and athletic and gymnastic abilities — because those skills understandably draw the attention of spectators and are easier to judge than internal aspects. While internal health and harmony provide the receiver with spectacular benefits, they aren't spectacular for spectators. I did my best to fight this trend, but after several years of swimming against the tide, I realised that the fundamental differences would always exist. I decided to resign from all of the positions and focus entirely on building Tai Chi for Health.

Soon I would find new inspiration for developing this new tai chi concept. I am so sensitive to motion that even watching waves on television makes me nauseous. On a trip to the United States I became so sick on the plane that by the time we touched down in Los Angeles I could hardly stand up. Eventually I found that surviving air travel meant keeping my eyes closed most of the time and practicing seated tai chi frequently.

One day in 1996 as I flew home from the US, I experienced a long period of soul-searching during the fourteen-hour flight. At one point a thought flashed through my mind. I had experienced arthritis since my early teens. As a family physician and acupuncturist, I possessed the qualifications to practice Western and traditional Chinese medicine. And I had extensive knowledge of the various styles of tai chi. Given all of this, it made sense for me to create a special tai chi program for individuals suffering with arthritis. This epiphany resulted in the beginning of the journey to what would eventually be called Tai Chi for Health. By the time the plane touched down in Sydney, I had chosen the style and forms for the Tai Chi for Arthritis program and worked out the steps.

As happens, once home I got swept up in work and life. A few weeks later, however, one of my long-time patients, Judith White, came in for an appointment. For several years I tried to talk Judith into learning tai chi to help her arthritis and hypertension. Judith told me that a few days prior to her appointment, she finally attended a tai chi class with her daughter. She didn't continue, however, because she felt the class too difficult for her, and she explained why.

During the first lesson, the teacher spent half an hour talking about tai chi theory while all of the students stood still. Fascinated at first, Judith became overwhelmed with the yin and yang and five element theories. Worse, standing for so long made her arthritic knees ache.

Judith wasn't the only one to complain to me about the ineffectiveness of tai chi classes. Many of my patients tried tai chi on my advice and gave up for similar reasons. Worse still, some with arthritis found that the lessons aggravated their condition. Some traditional teachers don't know how to teach tai chi effectively and fail to safely instruct people with chronic conditions like arthritis.

Judy's experience fuelled my enthusiasm for developing a tai chi program for arthritis and an accompanying video. I realised that not only did we need a safe, effective and easy-to-learn tai chi program but that the teaching methodology badly needed modernisation. Much of new research on learning had by that time unearthed more effective teaching methods.

Over the years, I've learned different aspects of tai chi and analysed them all medically — from traditional forms and their martial arts aspects to competition forms. I discovered that the secret to tai chi is the principles. No matter what form and style of tai chi you do, the principles — control of movement, good body structure, your internal state of mind, breathing, weight transference, and situation awareness — are the same. Tai chi principles are the core values derived from the collective wisdom of many tai chi experts. Every single tai chi movement incorporates most, if not all, of the principles, which means a tai chi set, no matter how short, can bring about the full power of tai chi. This constituted our basis for constructing the Tai Chi for Health programs. We used only twelve Sun style movements for Tai Chi for Arthritis, yet it incorporates all of the tai chi principles and delivers many benefits to the mind and the body in a relatively short period of time.

Later, it took the greater part of a year to recruit a highly qualified medical and tai chi team, testing and composing the program; and more time to construct instructional material including a step by step video teaching the first Tai Chi for Health instructor training workshop. All of my prior training in tai chi, medicine and teaching and my life experience prepared me for the task, however. When I realised that I could share the healing power of tai chi with people experiencing many different types of medical conditions, I created Tai Chi for Health as an overall umbrella for the various programs. In addition to the Tai Chi for Arthritis program, I developed Tai Chi for Diabetes, Osteoporosis, Back Pain and others, all with the same objective and using similar training methods.

Soon people wanted even more. I responded by explaining that tai chi possesses indefinite depth, and it isn't about how many movements you learn. Tai chi is an internal art that integrates mind and body, cultivating internal energy, and promoting health and harmony. The flowing movements of tai chi contain much inner strength, like water flowing in a river. Beneath the tranquil surface there is a current with immense power — the power for healing and wellness. So, for example, Tai Chi for Arthritis, though a short set, offers all that is needed to develop your internal energy and health and bring your tai chi to as high a level as you wish.

With consistent practice, people will be able to feel the internal energy (*qi*), convert it to internal force (*jing*), and use it to generate more internal energy. This process would greatly enhance tai chi development. After explaining this, I realised the need to show people how to access the *qi* and *jing*, so in 2002 I created my "Exploring the Depth of Tai Chi for Arthritis" workshop. It became my most popular, and I've conducted it hundreds of times around the world, with over ten thousand participants.

I distilled the essential tai chi principles from many years of studies and practice and translated them into plain language that focuses on the body's internal components, structure, and outward movements. *Song* and *jing* are the key internal components. *Song* refers to loosening or gently expanding from within all joints. This loosening then leads to strengthening the joints and relaxation of the mind. *Jing*, when used with tai chi, represents mental quietness or serenity and being mindful of the present. Both *song* and *jing* are most powerful at cultivating *qi*.

The body structure consists of correct alignment and weight transfer. Controlling all tai chi movements to be slow, smooth and continuous stretches and exercises the entire body and enhances the *jing* and *song*. Moving gently against mild resistance develops internal strength.

Translating the principles into easy-to-understand language and practical movements allows participants to experience them. All principles have many layers of depth and as we climb the tai chi mountain the air gets fresher and the view more beautiful.

Coming
Full Circle

*With time and patience the mulberry leaf
becomes a silk gown.*
CHINESE PROVERB

Recent journeys I've made back home to China have brought my life full circle. I have brought close members of my Tai Chi for Health family with me to visit the village where I grew up and my boarding school in Chaozhou. They saw the little storage room Aunt and I called home. Most importantly, they met my Chinese family — Zheng's children and grandchildren. The harmony and energy created by my two families fusing into one have stirred emotions of gratitude and wonder deep in my heart.

I escaped China as a teenager in a journey fraught with danger. If we'd been caught, there would have been no second chance. I never dreamed that I would freely return on my own terms with people from different parts of the world. Yet there I stood, a mature and successful physician, teacher of tai chi and researcher, travelling back in time with my tai chi family from many countries to show them the wonders of China — not only for my own entertainment and edification, but to broaden their perspectives and improve their skills.

Since 2000, myself and master trainers taught by me have trained more than 25,000 instructors globally. More than five million people are practicing my program every day. Arthritis foundations, user organisations and governmental departments around the world support my programs, including the US Centers for Disease Control and Prevention (www.CDC.gov). Of all the countries where I've spread the Tai Chi for Health vision, Singapore is one of my favourites, but it proved challenging to enter. I have great admiration for Singapore. The people are friendly, honest, hardworking and self-driven, and the government is efficient and caring. Singapore demonstrates that different races and cultures can coexist harmoniously and successfully. Most of the people are Chinese, which makes me proud that the Chinese culture could incubate and sustain an exceptional community for all citizens to grow and enjoy.

The culture of working hard does bring some negativity however. Singaporeans often become highly stressed from the pressure within and outside themselves. I have great affinity for them because I am also obsessed with cleanliness and working hard. Tai chi is an excellent antidote for the pressure brought on by hard work as it brings balance badly needed at times of extreme challenge.

It did not matter how much I liked Singapore or how hard and how many times I tried, nothing happened for many years until April 2, 2007. I received an e-mail from the country's chairman of the National Arthritis Foundation, Professor P. H. Feng, referring to the Tai Chi for Arthritis study that had been published in *Arthritis Care & Research*. Impressed at how the study showed that practicing tai chi relieves arthritis pain and improves the ability to perform daily activities, Professor Feng invited me to conduct a public talk and an instructors' training workshop.

Events moved quickly from there. Professor Feng introduced me to Professor Raymond Lau, who has a personal interest in tai chi. He became my translator and assisted me with what would be many packed instructor training workshops and public lectures. Professor Lau lectures at the National University of Singapore and is a rheumatologist and a visionary person. We became good friends, shared many ideas and stimulated each other's thinking.

One day he said to me, "For just about every important matter in life there is a simple, common truth that would be universal. Knowing that common truth would give us a clear direction to understand how everything works." I have always thought in a similar way. There is a simple common core truth at the heart of every art and science. I find it in life everywhere. For example, certain core values of human nature like love and the need to be loved apply to anyone from any country and culture. The essential tai chi principles hold true in so many aspects of life.

In May 2010, on the occasion of Singapore's Wellness Day I was invited to hold a teaching session at the headquarters of the People's Association, a department of the Singapore government. My tai chi colleagues and friends rallied together to help me prepare for the event, which they initially thought would draw 400 people. To everyone's surprise, so many people wanted to come that they had to cut off attendance at 2,000.

They planned the event for the early morning hours, because Singapore weather is too hot past 9 a.m. for older adults to exercise outdoors. Precisely at 8 a.m., 45 buses brought in 2,000 participants, who went through security and lined up by 8:30 a.m., with every twenty persons assigned to one Tai Chi for Health instructor. The planning resembled a military operation; I don't think such precision and timing could be accomplished in any other country.

When I walked onstage at precisely 9 a.m., the cheers suddenly sounded like jeers and threw me back all those years to the Midnight Terrors. Just as quickly, my tai chi training pulled me into the present. Without missing a step, I embraced the good will and positive energy of the audience and proceeded to share the excitement and power of tai chi.

As I looked out at the sea of smiling faces on that monumental morning, I experienced an overwhelming joy knowing that Aunt would have been so proud of me.

Afterword

I shake my head sometimes and wonder how a deprived, starving child from a little Chinese village ended up empowering millions to improve their health. On deep reflection, one theme stands out. In those difficult early years filled with potentially cataclysmic events, my aunt showered me with unconditional love that saved me from destruction. Love gave my life value and formed a firm foundation from which I developed inner strength. The bond between Aunt and I gave us the will to fight against all odds to survive the Great Famine.

Challenges that did not crush me made me grow in strength and skill. Rising from "down under" kindled my fighting spirit. The Empty Period taught me to embrace every opportunity. I learned to cope with culture shock in Hong Kong and Australia and appreciate the best each had to offer.

With my training in Western and Chinese medicine, as the Tai Chi for Health vision grew, I realised I possessed the opportunity and skills to bridge the gaps between Eastern and Western culture and modernise traditional tai chi, making it accessible to everyone. My arthritis, though painful, proved a blessing in disguise as it motivated me to practice and develop a program to help others. As if organised by a powerful underlying force, my unique combination of skills enabled me to conceive and lead the Tai Chi for Health vision.

The modern world is a stressful place, and I increasingly realize how much Tai Chi for Health can do — not just for chronic conditions but for everyone. Self-management and prevention is the best, if not the only way for the future. To enable people to proactively pursue health and wellness, we created Tai Chi for Beginners and Tai Chi for Energy. Later we built yet another bridge, Tai Chi for Rehabilitation, to help everyone from the simply tired and burned out to those with major health challenges to recover and follow a path to better health and wellness.

Reaching millions proved just the beginning. With the Tai Chi for Health Institute, my colleagues can take over. Our instructors and participants can pass on the baton, helping society reconnect with nature and themselves, improve relationships, and maybe even help make the earth more sustainable for the human race.

I embrace every challenge and love finding ways to listen to and redirect the incoming force. When I practice tai chi, I feel strong and serene from within. I relish my increasing strength and flexibility and value the serenity that tai chi gives me. Words cannot describe the overwhelming sense of fulfilment and happiness when I hear from people whom I have never met that I have changed their lives for the better. Any energy I expend on my mission is returned to me many times over.

In 2013, I retired from my medical practice. I continue to be involved in medical research and regard myself as a doctor, but now I practice preventative medicine full time. The world is my waiting room and my potential patients are everywhere. With the help of my tai chi colleagues, the size of my practice is unlimited.

I wasn't sure if I was ready for retirement but now I realise that I haven't retired, simply refocused. My excitement and energy is unbounded as I devote the rest of my life to the Tai Chi for Health vision. I hope you will join me on my journey and that one day our paths will cross.

My Recipe
for Health

I enjoy analysing all of the factors of a problem and devising a formula to solve it. Using this method to understand how the body and mind function, I worked out Tai Chi for Health programs that help people function in more effective and fulfilling ways. I am thrilled when I discover just the right therapy to solve a person's health challenge.

Ultimately, I love to find a solution to empower people to achieve better health and wellness. I talk to my patients, friends, tai chi colleagues and participants of my workshops about this topic frequently. Here is a recipe for health that works for me and many of the people with whom I've interacted. Most of these are woven into this book.

THE INGREDIENTS:
- *Positivity*
- *Responsibility*
- *Activity*
- *Engagement*
- *Interaction*

1. Positivity
Though it's human nature to highlight the negative, I always try to focus on the positive or bright side. Focusing

on difficulties may help us work harder during disasters, but in normal times, negativity can adversely affect our health, thinking and relationships. By looking for the best qualities in people, I enhance my relationships with them. Everyone likes to be recognised, which bolsters their confidence, resulting in more positive attitudes that lead to more win-win situations.

Whenever I feel down, I remind myself to "*song*" my joints — a tai chi state of gently loosening the joints, thus strengthening the body, inducing serenity and reminding me to stand tall. I may not feel great, but that simple change in posture tricks my mind into feeling less stressed and thinking more upright.

Even during really bad times, being sad does not make matters any better. I find psychologists are helpful when they advise that if you can't be happy, pretend to be, and soon you will be. Even if I can't be happy, it's best to avoid focusing on sadness.

2. Responsibility

I realised in my twenties that I needed to take responsibility for my own health. With crippling arthritis, I could have relied entirely on drugs to keep me relatively pain free. It took dedication to establish a major improvement through tai chi, but on the way I learned that keeping physically and mentally balanced in life provides the best way to cope with arthritis, as well as most matters in life.

As I mature, I take more responsibility for my actions. Whenever something goes wrong, I make an effort not to blame the circumstances and other people — not even the weather. Blaming anything or anyone, including myself, when something goes wrong fails to help me get to a better place. Blame might soothe my insecurity for a little while, but it wastes time and prevents healing. I find it more helpful to focus on analysing a situation rationally and looking at what was done and what can be improved. My best line of defence is developing inner strength, which reduces my insecurity.

I've also learned to be responsible for my reaction to other's actions. For example, when someone makes a racially discriminative remark, I hold my anger and make a great effort to keep my mind balanced. If that person means to upset me and I become angry, he or she controls me. If the person made an innocent mistake, I would have gotten upset for no reason. Worse still, an angry reaction would harm my relationship with that person. It is my responsibility to stay calm and find the most rational way to deal with life events.

3. Activity

Move it or lose it. If "it" equals physical ability, then I certainly have kept moving it, and I'm far from losing it. I'm now fitter, more flexible and stronger than many people half my age. I truly enjoy gaining more strength and flexibility as I become older, instead of getting weaker and stiffer. Even more so, I enjoy the continual personal growth that tai chi gives me. I find excuses to be active. For example, if I forget something in my study on the third floor, I don't wait to accumulate all of the things I have forgotten. I immediately walk up to the study to fetch it. I find excuses to practice tai chi whenever I can. If someone asks me to show them some tai chi, that provides an excellent excuse to practice.

4. Engagement

I fully immerse myself in most things I do — from my morning practice to working in my office to enjoying an excellent meal with friends. By engaging with activities, goals and relationships, I feel I'm truly living my life. One of my patients told me that he would do a day's work, come home and not remember anything he had done. The work proved too boring to engage him. He responded by changing his job.

If I'm just doing something to kill time, I am wasting life's most precious gift, and I'm not fully living. I would rather be engaging with a venture, like producing a video, even if it turns out not as well as expected. Not venturing is not living my life as fully as I could. We learn from every experience. The same holds true for relationships. By engaging with others, I gain happiness and excitement that I wouldn't experience without being fully present. I love "having a go" at so many things.

5. Interaction

Studies show that interacting with a lot of people increases our immunity. I have friends all over the globe and take an interest in their culture, views and personal stories. I strive to make my relationships with others as positive as possible. I take the same stance when representing our group to the community. I have an interest in conservation and the future of our planet and have been taking steps to make my workshops and business environmentally friendly. Though apolitical, I have a keen interest in our democratic system. I firmly believe that the tai chi community has a role to play in the health and well-being of our community and the planet.

A GOOD WAY TO COOK IT UP

Once I make a decision to proactively take control of my health, I feel better immediately. As I proceed with implementing my decision, every step makes me feel more in control and confident. When I overcome the inertia and persist with regular use of these ingredients, I feel even better. Feeling good about myself is the key to mental health.

From my lifelong learning, I've found that medical advances on health improvement correlate well with the ancient art of tai chi. Tai Chi for Health is an effective tool to enhance all of these five ingredients and helps to put them together in a balanced and harmonious way, like a good chef masterfully combining ingredients.

- By maintaining an upright posture, we "*song*" the joints, especially the spine, which facilitates a positive mind-set. Tai chi principles emphasise physical and mental balance with more positivity balancing out the human nature of being negative.
- Tai chi trains us to control our movements, improve our balance, and achieve serenity of mind or *jing*. This controlled training leads to freedom to move better with greater flexibility. More mobility from improved balance and a more

balanced mind lead to thinking more freely. In turn that enhances responsibility for our health and actions.

- Tai chi is an ideal activity that not only stretches, exercises and strengthens all muscles, ligaments, joints and internal organs, it also exercises the mind.
- Tai chi is meditation in motion; it facilitates engaging your body and mind, and leads to more mental tranquillity.
- Tai chi principles teach us how to interact with others more positively and effectively. By listening to the incoming force, we understand others better. By absorbing the incoming force, we can better redirect others to a win-win solution, thus establishing positive person-to person-relationships. The same rationale can improve interaction between one group of people and another. If a country listens to another, there might be no war.

Tai chi is based on nature and provides many natural ways to conserve our environment. To practice and experience health benefits, there is no need for equipment or to burn carbon.

Practicing Tai Chi for Health offers all of these healthful ingredients. So have a go!

A Tai Chi Sampler

While health and fitness benefits from tai chi can come relatively quickly, tai chi requires good instruction and regular practice. Discovering the depth of tai chi can be a journey of a lifetime. However, just to get a feel for what it's like to practice tai chi, try these exercises.

The Dan Tian Breathing Method

This breathing method was created based on traditional qigong and modern medical research. Dan tian is a Chinese word for the body's centre of energy or *qi*. It is located three fingers-width below your belly button and three fingers-width inside. The area is your centre of gravity and the storage house of qi, your life energy.

The breathing method enables you to sink and cultivate your qi to the dan tian, in turn improving internal energy. It can be incorporated into all qigong and tai chi movements.

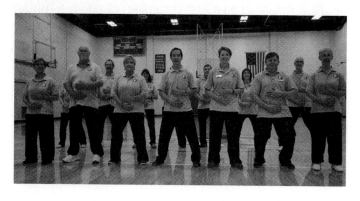

You can practise the breathing either sitting or standing upright. Be aware of using good posture. To get a feel for the practice, place your left hand on your abdomen just above the belly button and right hand below it. Focus on your lower abdomen and the pelvic floor muscle.

When you inhale, expand your lower abdominal area — allow it to bulge out a little gently — and let your abdominal and pelvic floor muscles relax. You should feel a slight pushing out of the right hand. As you exhale, gently contract the pelvic floor muscles and the lower abdomen. Feel the contraction of the muscles with your right hand, keeping the area above your belly button as still as possible. Contract the pelvic floor muscles very gently, so gently that it's almost like you're just thinking about contracting them.

Another approach is simply to imagine that you're bringing your pelvic floor just half an inch closer to your belly button. A stronger contraction would move the left hand too much and that would involve different groups of muscles and therefore not be as effective.

As you inhale and relax the pelvic and lower abdominal muscles, try not to relax them completely but retain approximately 10–20 per cent of the contraction. This will allow you to maintain an upright posture and have the right group of muscles ready for the next phase.

Once you have become familiar with this technique, you don't have to place your hands on the abdomen. Simply do the breathing exercise and maintain an upright posture (even when sitting). You can get a free video lesson on how to do this exercise and learn more about its medical implications:

http://www.taichiproductions.com/dvds/health/
tai-chi-for-rehabilitation-empowering-people-to-well-
ness-free-first-lesson/

The Posture of Opening and Closing

In this qigong exercise, begin by standing upright with your feet shoulder-width apart. Look straight ahead. Tuck in your chin and relax your shoulders, elbows and knees. Imagine your body as a string that is being stretched gently from both ends. Be mindful of your relaxed, upright posture.

1. As you inhale, slowly bring your hands up, arms extended, to chest height, palms facing each other.
2. Bring your hands toward your chest bending your knees slightly.
3. Inhale and slowly pull your hands apart to shoulder width.

As you exhale, push your hands toward each other, bringing them as close to each other as possible without touching. Slowly open and close your hands several times, again inhaling as you separate your hands, exhaling as you close them.

As you breathe in and out, imagine there is a gentle magnetic force between your palms. Pull against the force as you breathe in and push against it as you breathe out. Try to do three repetitions.

Complete the exercise by stretching your hands forward then bringing them back to your side and straightening your knees.

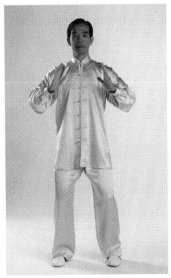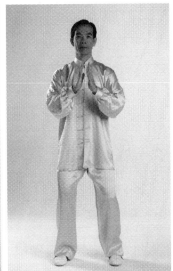

For another challenge, try combining the dan tian breathing method with the posture of opening and closing. As you open your hands, breathe in and relax your lower abdomen, and as you close your hands, breathe out and contract your lower abdomen.

To learn more, take a free video lesson:

http://www.taichiproductions.com/dvds/health/tai-chi-for-rehabilitation-empowering-people-to-wellness-free-first-lesson/

Single Whip

1. Start with the above opening and closing position. Slowly open your hands, feeling the gentle resistance and breathing in. Close your hands, pushing gently against the resistance and breathing out.

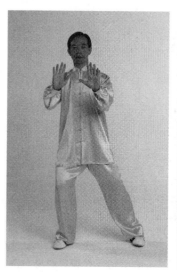 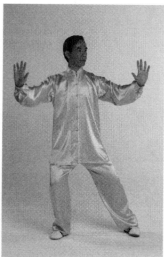

2. After open and close, transfer your weight to the right foot and then lift the left foot up, placing it to the left and slightly forward. Keep your body upright. Move your hands forward, shifting your weight forward. Turn your palms outward, weight forward.

3. Open up your hands as if you were opening up a set of curtains. Your right hand moves a little faster than the left. As you open up your palms, turn your torso slightly to the right, looking at your right hand.

4. Finish by returning to the open and close position. Open and close your hands. Extend your hands forward, lower your arms back to your side, and bring your feet back together.

Resources

FREE TAI CHI LESSONS ON YOUTUBE

A great way to get started with tai chi is to check out the various videos offered online by Dr. Lam. Search "Paul Lam free tai chi lesson" on YouTube and the search results will produce links to Tai Chi for Health lessons of various styles, including *Tai Chi for Beginners*. This video, which has received well over four million views on YouTube, provides an excellent introduction to tai chi, as well as a free first lesson. If you find it appealing, you can order the DVD for the full set of lessons, or begin lessons with a certified Tai Chi for Health Instructor.

Direct link to Tai Chi for Beginners introduction and free lesson: http://youtu.be/hIOHGrYCEJ4.

To search for a certified Tai Chi for Health instructor near you, visit: www.taichihealthinstitute.com.

TAI CHI FOR HEALTH INSTITUTE

The Tai Chi for Health Institute (www.taichiforhealth.org), a nonprofit organisation founded by Dr. Paul Lam, is an educational institute regarding all aspect of the Tai Chi for Health programs. It set up curriculum and training for all levels of instructors and monitors the quality and standard of all instructors. It also offers an array of information for getting started with tai chi, or extending your practice. Find info on tai chi workshops, instructors, videos, books, tai chi philosophy and history and more. The site hosts links to free lessons on health and tai chi. TCHI is an excellent starting point for learning what tai chi can do for you and how you can get involved in the global tai chi community.

Sign up for a weekly newsletter to keep abreast of tai chi news, workshops and events.

TAI CHI PRODUCTIONS

Dr. Paul Lam's company, Tai Chi Productions (www.taichiproductions.com), is dedicated to advancing the Tai Chi for Health Programs through research, education and instruction. The website offers an array of tai chi materials, including downloadable lessons, instructional DVDs, books, music CDs and more. *Tai Chi for Beginners — 8 Lessons*, also the *Tai Chi for Arthritis program — 12 lessons* is available here as individual downloadable lessons or as a video program. Another popular starting point is the book *Tai Chi for Beginners and the 24 Forms*. A wide variety of instructional materials for intermediate and advanced tai chi programs are also available on the website.

NEWSLETTER

Subscribe to Dr. Lam's monthly newsletter to receive regular personal observations by Dr. Lam on tai chi issues and to follow reports on his travels worldwide in teaching tai chi. Contributors include Tai Chi for Health master trainers and other tai chi experts. Students often chime in with testimonials about how they have improved their health and lives through tai chi.

Subscribe at http://www.taichiforhealthinstute.org/ newsletters/healthinstute.org/newsletters/.

FACEBOOK

Follow Tai Chi for Health on Facebook to keep up to date on tai chi workshops, events, videos and more. Also, find updates on newsletters, research news and videos. Dr. Lam also enjoys posting some of his favorite tai chi photos from his travels around the world.

Visit www.facebook.com/taichihealth/.

WORLD TAI CHI & QIGONG DAY

Visit www.worldtaichiday.org to learn about this annual global celebration of tai chi, held on the last Saturday in April. Tai chi and qigong practitioners come together from more than 80 nations to "breathe together, providing a healing vision for our world". The website also contains information on "all things tai chi and qigong". It includes a teacher's directory, medical research on tai chi, learning tips and more.

BOOKS

You can purchase Dr Lam's other books (also in eBook format) at www.taichiproductions.com, including these ones below.

Teaching Tai Chi Effectively

Dr Lam, one of the most experienced and respected tai chi teachers in the world, shares practical and proven methods to make tai chi accessible to everyone. This book contains useful material for any tai chi teacher, including working with people of different ages and conditions from arthritis to Parkinson's, pregnant women to older adults. Thousands of teachers have adopted his methods, resulting in dramatic increase in retention rates and greater student and teacher enjoyment.

Tai Chi for Beginners & the 24 Forms
Contains step-by-step instructions and photographs of Six Easy Steps for Beginners and the 24 Forms. It contains a wide range of relevant information and helps you develop your tai chi to higher levels.

Born Strong
The Tai Chi Way is based on a larger work, Dr Lam's memoir. If you enjoyed this bookazine, you might wish to read *Born Strong*, which offers more episodes from Dr Lam's dramatic life and deeper insights into tai chi and personal development.